Questions and Answers About Overactive Bladder and Urinary Incontinence

Pamela Ellsworth
Chief, Division of Urology
University of Massachusetts
Memorial Medical Center
Worcester, MA

David A. Gordon
University of Maryland
Medical Director
Chesapeake Urology Center for
Continence and Pelvic Floor Disorders
Owings Mills, MD

with
Jennifer Bagdigian

JONES AND BARTLETT PUBLISHERS
Sudbury, Massachusetts
BOSTON   TORONTO   LONDON   SINGAPORE

World Headquarters

Jones and Bartlett
Publishers
40 Tall Pine Drive
Sudbury, MA 01776
info@jbpub.com
www.jbpub.com

Jones and Bartlett
Publishers Canada
2406 Nikanna Road
Mississauga, ON L5C 2W6
CANADA

Jones and Bartlett
Publishers International
Barb House, Barb Mews
London W6 7PA
UK

Jones and Bartlett's books and products are available through most bookstores and online booksellers. To contact Jones and Bartlett Publishers directly, call 800-832-0034, fax 978-443-8000, or visit our website www.jbpub.com.

Substantial discounts on bulk quantities of Jones and Bartlett's publications are available to corporations, professional associations, and other qualified organizations. For details and specific discount information, contact the special sales department at Jones and Bartlett via the above contact information or send an email to specialsales@jbpub.com.

The authors, editor, and publisher have made every effort to provide accurate information. However, they are not responsible for errors, omissions, or for any outcomes related to the use of the contents of this book and take no responsibility for the use of the products described. Treatments and side effects described in this book may not be applicable to all patients; likewise, some patients may require a dose or experience a side effect that is not described herein. The reader should confer with his or her own physician regarding specific treatments and side effects. Drugs and medical devices are discussed that may have limited availability controlled by the Food and Drug Administration (FDA) for use only in a research study or clinical trial. The drug information presented has been derived from reference sources, recently published data, and pharmaceutical research data. Research, clinical practice, and government regulations often change the accepted standard in this field. When consideration is being given to use of any drug in the clinical setting, the health care provider or reader is responsible for determining FDA status of the drug, reading the package insert, reviewing prescribing information for the most up-to-date recommendations on dose, precautions, and contraindications, and determining the appropriate usage for the product. This is especially important in the case of drugs that are new or seldom used.

Production Credits
Chief Executive Officer: Clayton Jones
Chief Operating Officer: Don W. Jones, Jr.
President, Higher Education and Professional Publishing: Robert W. Holland, Jr.
V.P., Sales and Marketing: William J. Kane
V.P., Design and Production: Anne Spencer
V.P., Manufacturing and Inventory Control: Therese Connell
Executive Publisher: Christopher Davis
Production Director: Amy Rose
Associate Production Editor: Dan Stone
Editorial Assistant: Kathy Richardson
Director of Marketing: Alisha Weisman
Marketing Associate: Laura Kavigian
Manufacturing and Inventory Coordinator: Amy Bacus
Composition: Northeast Compositors, Inc.
Cover Design: Kate Ternullo
Cover Image: © Photodisc
Printing and Binding: Malloy, Inc.
Cover Printing: Malloy, Inc.

Library of Congress Cataloging-in-Publication Data
Ellsworth, Pamela.
    Questions & answers about overactive bladder and urinary incontinence
/ Pamela Ellsworth, David A. Gordon, and Jennifer Bagdigian. -- Special sale ed.
      p. cm.
    Abridged ed. of: 100 questions & answers about overactive bladder
and urinary incontinence.
    ISBN 0-7637-3934-0
    1. Urinary incontinence--Popular works. 2. Bladder--Diseases--Popular
works. 3. Bladder--Popular works.   I. Gordon, David A., MD.
II. Ellsworth, Pamela. 100 questions & answers about overactive bladder
and urinary incontinence. III. Title. IV. Title: Questions and answers
about overactive bladder and urinary incontinence.
RC921.I5.E433 2006
616.6'2--dc22
                                        2005025301

Printed in the United States of America
09 08 07 06 05   10 9 8 7 6 5 4 3 2 1

Contents

Overactive bladder (OAB) and urinary incontinence affect over 30 million male and female Americans. The risk of developing overactive bladder increases with age in both males and females. These conditions, overactive bladder and urinary incontinence, are associated with a significant negative impact on quality of life and such medical problems as urinary tract infections, skin irritation, and, in the elderly, an increased risk of falls and fractures. Urinary incontinence is responsible for nearly 50% of nursing home admissions. There is a huge economic impact of these conditions also. Continence supplies, such as diapers and pads, are only a portion of the healthcare dollars spent on these conditions.

YET, despite the high prevalence, the significant effects on quality of life, the associated medical morbidities and the financial impact of these conditions, they remain largely undiagnosed and untreated. WHY is this the case? Unfortunately, there are several barriers to the identification and treatment of these conditions on both the part of the patient and the physician. Sufferers of these conditions may believe that (1) the condition(s) is an inevitable part of aging, an incorrect assumption; (2) the condition is too embarrassing to discuss with the physician; (3) the symptoms are "minor" compared to those of their friends/family with "life-threatening" illnesses and thus they trivialize their own problems; and (4) there is no effective treatment, again an incorrect assumption. Some individuals may bring the subject up with their doctors but receive no evaluation or treatment. A validated screening tool, the OAB-V8, has been developed to help identify individuals with overactive bladder. In addition, physicians will often wait for the patient to bring up the problem, which, as stated, is often difficult for the patient to do. Once the situation is noted, there is often a lack of evaluation and treatment. Lastly, the management of overactive bladder and urinary incontinence is continually evolving and physicians need to be aware of the newer therapies in order to best counsel patients.

Many of these limitations to the evaluation and management of overactive bladder and urinary incontinence are a result of the lack of knowledge about these conditions. It is our sincere hope that this book provides knowledge to empower OAB and urinary incontinence sufferers to seek help and to be actively involved in their management plan so that their quality of life and medical health may be improved. If we can touch the lives of even a few OAB and urinary incontinence sufferers, we will have achieved our goal. Read on and find out how you can take control of a problem(s) that has taken control of your life.

OAB-V8
Overactive Bladder-**Validated** 8-question Awareness Tool[1]

The questions below ask about how bothered you may be by some bladder symptoms. Some people are bothered by bladder symptoms and may not realize that there are treatments available for their symptoms. Please circle that number that best describes how much you have been bothered by each symptom. Add the numbers together for a total score and record the score in the box provided at the bottom.

How bothered have you been by...	Not at all	A little bit	Some-what	Quite a bit	A great deal	A very great deal
1. Frequent urination during the daytime hours?	0	1	2	(3)	4	5
2. An uncomfortable urge to urinate?	0	1	2	3	(4)	5
3. A sudden urge to urinate with little or no warning?	0	1	2	3	(4)	5
4. Accidental loss of small amounts of urine?	0	1	(2)	3	4	5
5. Nighttime urination?	0	(1)	2	3	4	5
6. Waking up at night because you had to urinate?	0	(1)	2	3	4	5
7. An uncontrollable urge to urinate?	0	1	2	3	4	(5)
8. Urine loss associated with a strong desire to urinate?	0	1	(2)	3	4	5
Are you a male?			If male, ☐ add 2 points to your score			

Please add up your responses to the questions above 2 2

Please hand this page to your healthcare provider when you see him/her for your visit.

If your score is 8 or greater, you may have overactive bladder. There are effective treatments for this condition. You may want to talk with a healthcare professional about your symptoms.

Note: You may be asked to give a urine sample. Please ask before going to the bathroom.

Reference: 1. Coyne KS, Zyczynski T, Margolis MK, Elinoff V, Roberts RG. Validation of an overactive bladder awareness tool for use in a primary care setting. *Adv Ther.* In press.

OAB-V8
Overactive Bladder-**Validated** 8-question Awareness Tool[1]

The questions below ask about how bothered you may be by some bladder symptoms. Some people are bothered by bladder symptoms and may not realize that there are treatments available for their symptoms. Please circle that number that best describes how much you have been bothered by each symptom. Add the numbers together for a total score and record the score in the box provided at the bottom.

How bothered have you been by...	Not at all	A little bit	Some-what	Quite a bit	A great deal	A very great deal
1. Frequent urination during the daytime hours?	0	1	2	3	4	5
2. An uncomfortable urge to urinate?	0	1	2	3	4	5
3. A sudden urge to urinate with little or no warning?	0	1	2	3	4	5
4. Accidental loss of small amounts of urine?	0	1	2	3	4	5
5. Nighttime urination?	0	1	2	3	4	5
6. Waking up at night because you had to urinate?	0	1	2	3	4	5
7. An uncontrollable urge to urinate?	0	1	2	3	4	5
8. Urine loss associated with a strong desire to urinate?	0	1	2	3	4	5

Are you a male?　　　　　　If male, ☐ add 2 points to your score

Please add up your responses to the questions above ☐☐

Please hand this page to your healthcare provider when you see him/her for your visit.

If your score is 8 or greater, you may have overactive bladder. There are effective treatments for this condition. You may want to talk with a healthcare professional about your symptoms.

Note: You may be asked to give a urine sample. Please ask before going to the bathroom.
Reference: 1. Coyne KS, Zyczynski T, Margolis MK, Elinoff V, Roberts RG. Validation of an overactive bladder awareness tool for use in a primary care setting. *Adv Ther.* In press.

PART ONE

The Basics

What is the bladder and what does it do?

What are normal voiding habits?

What problems can occur with bladder function?

More . . .

1. What is the bladder and what does it do?

The bladder is a hollow organ shaped like a sphere. It is designed to accomplish two jobs: (1) store urine at low pressures, and (2) when it is full, empty the urine. For the bladder to do this, it must be able to stretch to hold increasing amounts of fluid (urine) at low pressure. The lining of the bladder (the **urothelium**) and the bladder muscle (the **detrusor**) work together to allow the bladder to stretch. When the bladder is full, the bladder muscle must be able to contract strongly and for a long enough time so that the bladder can be completely emptied. The normal adult bladder holds around 10 to 15 ounces.

The kidneys produce urine constantly. Urine passes down the **ureter**, which is a long, thin, hollow tube that drains into the bladder. The wall of the ureter has muscle fibers that contract and relax, pushing urine down and into the bladder. This contraction of the ureter, along with gravity, helps ensure that urine moves from the kidney into the bladder. If bladder pressure is too high, the ureter can't push urine into the bladder. This causes a backup of urine, called **stasis**, within the ureter. If the backup continues, it can affect the kidney as well. To avoid this backup, the bladder must be "compliant" while it is storing urine. That is, it must be able to store urine at a low pressure until the bladder is full. When the bladder is full the muscle contracts, raising the bladder pressure. This leads to urination.

Once someone becomes toilet-trained, bladder emptying becomes voluntary. As the bladder fills, the **bladder outlet**—the area where the bladder joins the **urethra**—

Urothelium

the inner lining of the urinary tract (kidneys, ureter, bladder).

Detrusor

the bladder muscle. Coordinated contraction of the detrusor and opening of the bladder outlet allows for normal urination.

Ureter

a long, thin, hollow tube that connects the kidneys to the bladder so that urine can pass out of the kidney and into the bladder.

Stasis

a circumstance in which high pressure in the bladder causes a backup of urine within the ureter and eventually the kidneys.

Bladder outlet

the area where the bladder joins the urethra.

Urethra

the canal leading from the bladder to the body's skin to discharge urine.

stays closed. This maintains **continence** while the bladder fills and stores urine. During **voiding** the bladder and urethra work together so that as the bladder contracts the bladder outlet opens. This releases the urine through the bladder outlet into the urethra. The **urethral sphincter**, a muscle that contracts to close the urethra, also relaxes during voiding to allow for the passage of urine through the urethra.

The nervous system controls urination and helps maintain control of urine. It has two parts: the central nervous system (the brain and spinal cord), and the peripheral nervous system (the nerves found in all of the other parts of the body). Signals are constantly flowing from one nerve to another, telling each cell in the body what to do and when to do it. Some of these signals are consciously done, like when you want to move an arm, and other signals are done without you knowing about them. These unconscious signals drive most of the complicated bodily functions, such as blood flow and breathing.

The **central nervous system** is responsible for starting or preventing urination. It is composed of the parasympathetic and sympathetic nervous systems. The sympathetic nervous system allows the bladder to hold urine by telling the bladder muscle to relax. Storage of urine is also aided by contraction of the bladder neck and the urethral sphincter muscle.

The **peripheral nervous system** is also involved in urination. It helps in the coordination of bladder contraction and urethral relaxation during normal voiding.

When the parasympathetic nerves are stimulated, a chemical called a neurotransmitter is released. This

Continence
the ability to retain urine and/or feces until a proper time for their elimination.

Void
to eliminate urine.

Urethral sphincter
a muscle that, when contracted, closes the urethra.

Central nervous system
nerves in the brain and spinal cord; responsible for starting or preventing urination.

Peripheral nervous system
nerves connecting in the body other than at the brain and spinal cord; responsible for the coordination of bladder contraction and urethral relaxation during normal voiding.

The Basics

Acetylcholine

a chemical released from certain nerves that attaches to a receptor in the bladder wall, causing the bladder to contract.

Muscarinic receptor

a receptor in the bladder for acetylcholine.

chemical, **acetylcholine**, then attaches to a receptor on the bladder wall. This series of events causes the bladder muscle to contract.

The receptors for acetylcholine are called **muscarinic receptors**. There are five different muscarinic receptors located in the body. In the bladder there are two: M2 and M3. Although most of the muscarinic receptors in the bladder are M2 receptors, it appears that the M3 receptor is the main receptor responsible for bladder contractions. It is believed that M2 receptors may have a role in conditions such as spinal cord injury and bladder outlet obstruction.

In some individuals, their bladder may be "too sensitive" and they don't have the appropriate early warning. Instead, they will experience a sudden onset of incontinence with little or no warning. The urge to void is a normal sensation which can become stronger if one chooses to hold off urinating. Urgency is not normal. It is a sudden compelling desire to void that is often difficult to defer and may be associated with leakage/incontinence.

2. What are normal voiding habits?

Urinary frequency

having to void eight times or more per day with normal intake of fluids.

Nocturia

having to wake from sleep at night to urinate after a day of normal fluid intake.

It is hard to say what "normal voiding habits" are. How often you urinate depends on what you drink, how much you drink, the medications that you take, and the situations that you are in. Typically, the average adult voids roughly every three to four hours while awake and can sleep through the night without having to urinate. Individuals who void more than eight times per day are believed to have **urinary frequency**. Those who get up at night to void have **nocturia**. Remember, though, that if you drink six cups of coffee in the morning, you will need to void frequently due to the diuretic effect of the caffeine. If you drink three quarts of fluid a day, you will need to urinate more than eight times in the day. Individuals who take diuretics—sometimes called "water pills"—may also have to urinate frequently because of the increased urine volume that the pills produce.

3. What problems can occur with bladder function?

Problems with bladder function affect one or both of the bladder's two main functions—storing and releasing urine.

Storage problems can result from a bladder with a small capacity, an overactive bladder, or a poorly compliant bladder. Emptying problems can be due to a bladder that doesn't contract well or that has an outlet obstruction.

Storage Problems

A **small capacity bladder** does not hold much urine. This may be due to fibrosis or scarring within the bladder, or from neurologic causes. A small capacity bladder loses its ability to stretch, so it cannot hold a normal amount of urine. With this condition, you tend to void more frequently. Some individuals may have a normal bladder but a heightened awareness of bladder filling, which leads to urinary frequency.

An **overactive bladder** occurs when the bladder muscle contracts at times when it should be relaxed. This leads to **urinary urgency** (a sudden desire to void that is often difficult to put off), frequency (voiding more

Small capacity bladder

a bladder that cannot hold much urine because of fibrosis, scarring, or neurological causes.

Overactive bladder

a condition caused by the bladder muscle (detrusor) contracting at times when it should be relaxed, with symptoms of urinary urgency and often with frequency and nocturia.

Urinary urgency

sudden compelling desire to urinate that often is difficult to put off.

than eight times per day), and possibly nocturia (waking at night one or more times to void). If the contraction is strong enough there may be a loss of urine. This loss of urine is called **urgency incontinence**.

A **poorly compliant bladder** holds urine at higher than normal bladder pressure. This elevated bladder pressure can affect the drainage of urine from the kidneys causing a backup of urine in the kidneys, and eventually kidney damage.

Emptying Problems

The bladder muscle must contract to empty the bladder. If there is an **obstruction** or blockage in the urethra, the bladder must be able to create a higher pressure to push urine past the obstruction. In some cases there may be **poor contractility** of the bladder. This means that the bladder muscle can't squeeze (contract) strongly enough and/or stay contracted long enough to completely empty the bladder. Poor bladder contractility may result from:

1. injury to the nerves that affect the bladder, such as in a spinal cord injury.

2. inherited conditions, such as spina bifida.

3. chronic overdistention (over-stretching) of the bladder.

4. severe long-term bladder outlet obstruction from such causes as enlargement of the prostate or failure of the sphincter muscle to relax.

5. medications that affect the bladder's ability to contract.

Poor contractility of the bladder leaves increasing amounts of urine in the bladder after voiding. This **"postvoid residual" urine** may lead to urinary tract

Urgency incontinence

unintended leakage or loss of urine associated with urgency.

Poorly compliant bladder

a bladder that holds urine at higher than normal pressures, which may cause poor emptying of the kidneys, a backup of urine in the kidneys, and eventually kidney damage.

Obstruction

blockage of outflow of urine from the bladder.

Poor contractility

a situation in which the bladder cannot generate and/or sustain the contraction well enough to completely empty out the urine.

Postvoid residual urine

the amount of urine left behind in the bladder after voiding; if elevated, may lead to urinary tract infection, bladder stones, further distention of the bladder, worsening of bladder functions, and can lead to dilation of the kidneys and ureter.

infections, bladder stones, further distention (over-stretching) of the bladder, worsening bladder function, and/or higher bladder pressures that cause swelling of the kidneys and ureter.

An **acontractile bladder** does not contract. This may occur suddenly, with no prior history of any troubles with urination. This is called acute **urinary retention**. When a bladder stops contracting it may also be part of a slowly progressive problem. You may or may not feel an urge to urinate and will not be able to urinate. It is very important to treat urinary retention because, over a period of time, it may lead to kidney damage.

Acontractile bladder
a bladder that does not contract.

Urinary retention
the inability to urinate on one's own.

4. Is there an age when one is most at risk for urinary incontinence?

The risk of **urinary incontinence**—the inability to control the discharge of urine—increases with age for both men and women. Unfortunately, because urinary incontinence is so common in older women, it is sometimes thought to be a normal and inevitable part of aging. This is not true!

Urinary incontinence
involuntary loss of urine.

Urinary incontinence affects about 20%–23% of women between 30 and 39 years of age. This percentage increases to 25%–30% in those who are 40 to 49 years of age, and then remains stable until ages 75 to 89. From ages 75 to 89 the percentage increases to 30%–32% . It increases again at 90 years of age, when incontinence affects about 35% of women.

In men, the rate of urinary incontinence increases from 0.7% at 50 to 59 years of age to 2.7% for those 60 to 69 years of age. The rate is 3.4% for those 70 years of age and older. Remember that even though the risk of developing an overactive bladder increases with age, it is not a "normal expected part of aging." Most importantly, it can be treated.

Stress urinary incontinence

involuntary loss of urine from mild or heavy exertion, such as during sneezing, coughing, or heavy lifting.

Mixed urinary incontinence

involuntary leakage of urine associated with urgency as well as with exertion (such as sneezing, coughing, or during heavy lifting).

Functional incontinence

a situation in which the bladder, urethra, and pelvic floor muscles are functioning properly, but physical or mental function prevents you from independently getting to the bathroom on time.

Chronic retention

longstanding increased amount of urine in the bladder (postvoid residual). May be associated with urinary incontinence (overflow incontinence).

5. Are there other causes of urinary incontinence besides urge incontinence?

Yes. **Stress urinary incontinence** is the involuntary loss of urine you experience when you exert yourself doing anything from sneezing or coughing to heavy lifting. (See Questions 44–48.) **Mixed urinary incontinence** is involuntary leaking with urgency combined with the leaking you get from exertion. **Functional incontinence** occurs when the bladder, urethra, and pelvic floor muscles are working fine, but physical or mental function makes it difficult or impossible for you to get to the bathroom on your own in time. **Chronic retention** may lead to leakage of urine when the bladder is overdistended (expanded beyond its elastic capacity). This usually is the result of an obstruction due to benign prostate enlargement in men, but may also result from neurologic diseases, poor bladder muscle function, or as a side effect of medications. **Temporary (transient) incontinence** may be caused by illness or medications that increase the volume of urine produced to the point where it interferes with normal function.

6. How can I tell the difference between incontinence associated with an overactive bladder (urge incontinence) and stress incontinence?

A review of symptoms and a physical exam will help you and your doctor to identify the cause of your leakage. Some women will have both stress and urge incontinence, so there may be more than one cause for the leakage. An assessment of the presence or absence of the symptoms listed in Table 1 will help you to identify the cause of the leakage.

For a woman, this appointment includes an examination of your **perineum**. During this part of the exam, you will be asked to strain/bear down (this is called Valsalva maneuver) and cough while the doctor watches for movement of the urethra (hypermobility) and leakage of urine. Hypermobility or leakage with a Valsalva maneuver means that you probably have stress urinary incontinence. Men rarely develop stress incontinence unless they have undergone prior prostate surgery, such as a **radical prostatectomy** for prostate

Temporary (transient) incontinence
leakage of urine caused by illness or medications that increase the volume of urine produced to the point where it interferes with normal urinary tract function.

Perineum
area between the thighs extending from the tail bone (coccyx) to the pubis (between the vulva and anus in a woman and the scrotum and anus in a man) and lying below the pelvic diaphragm.

Radical prostatectomy
a surgical procedure to remove the entire prostate as treatment for prostate cancer.

The Basics

Table 1   Symptoms found in overactive bladder and stress incontinence

Symptoms	Overactive Bladder	Stress Incontinence
Urgency	Yes	No
Frequency with urgency	Yes	No
Leakage with physical activity (cough, laugh, sneeze)	No	Yes
Amount of urine leaked with each episode	Large, if present	Usually small
Ability to reach toilet in time following an urge to void	No or just barely	Yes
Need to wake up at night to urinate	Often	Not often

Transurethral prostatectomy (TURP)

removal of part of the prostate through the urethra.

Urodynamic study

a special test used to determine how the bladder and urethral muscles work; includes measuring storage and empty- ing of the bladder.

cancer or a **transurethral prostatectomy (TURP)** for benign enlargement of the prostate.

7. *What is a urodynamic study?*

A **urodynamic study** is a test that helps your doctor determine how your bladder and urethral muscles are working. This test looks at how well your bladder holds and then empties urine. It also looks at how well the urethra functions. A urodynamic study is helpful in diagnosing the type of incontinence you have, but is not necessary for everyone. Often this test is reserved for people who are not getting better on medical ther- apy and those who are thinking about having surgery.

There are several parts to a urodynamic study. Depending on your concerns, you may need some or all of the parts of the study.

The first part of a urodynamic study is often a "**uroflow**." In this test, you simply urinate into a con- tainer that measures how fast you urinate.

Uroflow

the rate of flow of the urine stream.

Filling cystometry

the part of the urody- namic study when the bladder is being filled and the pres- sures within the bladder are being measured.

After the uroflow study a **filling cystometry** is per- formed. For this test, a sterile catheter is placed into your bladder. The catheter is connected to a tube that allows sterile dye to be placed into your bladder and it is also connected to a pressure-monitoring device. Your bladder is then filled with the sterile dye and the pressure monitor notes changes in your bladder pres- sure. In addition, it assesses bladder sensation and compliance of the ability of the bladder to hold urine at a low pressure. The doctor may also take x-ray pic- tures, called **fluoroscopy**, to see how your bladder looks. If your doctor thinks you have stress inconti- nence, at times during the test he or she will ask you to strain by pushing out with your abdomen, bearing

Fluoroscopy

a type of x-ray that allows the doctor to see the tissues and deep structures of the body.

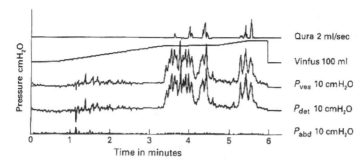

Figure 1   Uninhibited contractions in a bladder. (Reprinted with permission from Blandy J, Fowler C: Urology, 2e, 1996. Chapter 24: Bladder Disorders of Junction. Copyright © Blackwell Science, Inc.)

down, or coughing. The pressure in your bladder during this period can be measured and your doctor will take x-rays to see if you are leaking and if your bladder and urethra are supported properly. (See Figure 1.)

When you have a strong desire to void during the test, the doctor will ask you to do so. At this time a **pressure flow study** can be performed. This study measures how fast you are voiding and the pressure within your bladder during voiding.

Pressure flow study

a study to determine whether there is any obstruction to the outflow of urine.

For some people, particularly those that may have a nerve-related cause to their leakage, the doctor may place small patches or needles (electrodes) around the anus. These electrodes allow the doctor to see how your pelvic floor muscles are working while your bladder fills and when you urinate.

Urodynamic studies are performed while you are awake so that you can tell your doctor when you first feel the urge to urinate, when the urge gets stronger, and whether you are leaking.

The Basics

PART TWO

Diagnosis of Overactive Bladder

What is overactive bladder (OAB)?

Are there medical conditions that may cause or mimic OAB?

What causes OAB?

More . . .

8. What is overactive bladder?

Having an overactive bladder (OAB) means that your bladder contracts at times other than when you want to void. Typically, when your bladder fills the bladder muscle remains relaxed in order to hold the urine, and then contracts when you want to void. A contraction of the bladder at a time other than voiding is called an involuntary bladder contraction. This type of contraction may be felt as a need to urinate and, if the contraction is strong enough and/or the pelvic floor muscles are weak, you will leak. This is urge incontinence. If these contractions occur frequently, then you will experience urinary frequency.

The symptoms of OAB include urgency with or without urge incontinence, and are often associated with frequency and nocturia:

- Urgency is the sudden compelling desire to void, which is often difficult to put off.
- Urgency incontinence is the involuntary loss of urine that is accompanied by or immediately preceded by urgency.
- Urinary frequency is the need to void more than eight times in a 24-hour period.
- Nocturia is when you wake up at night one or more times to void.

Nocturia is very common. The likelihood of having it increases with age, and if you have it the symptoms may get worse as you get older. Although nocturia is common with OAB, it has several other causes. Your doctor will review your history and medications and may ask you to fill out a frequency volume chart. This chart (also called a bladder diary) helps your doctor determine the cause of your nocturia. (See also Question 13.)

9. What causes overactive bladder, and is it hereditary?

The main cause of overactive bladder isn't well known. Overactivity of the bladder may be related to a problem with nerves or a problem with the bladder muscle itself, among other causes. The central nervous system, which consists of the brain and the spinal cord, controls bladder function like an on-off circuit that you are able to voluntarily control. Damage to certain areas of the brain and spinal cord may alter this on-off circuit and lead to bladder overactivity. Neurological conditions that may be related to overactive bladder include Parkinson's disease, multiple sclerosis, and spinal cord injury. Conditions that may lead to changes in bladder muscle function include bladder outlet obstruction, such as in men with benign enlargement of the prostate gland (BPH), or aging. Urodynamic studies (discussed in Question 7) have shown that as we age, the bladder decreases in size. In addition, as we age there is an increased incidence of uninhibited bladder contractions, a decreased force of the urine stream, and a decreased volume of urine voided along with incomplete bladder emptying. Changes in the muscarinic receptors in the bladder may also occur with aging. Some aspects of diet and lifestyle may be associated with an increased risk of developing overactive bladder. These factors include drinking caffeinated soda, being overweight or obese, and smoking.

Lastly, changes in the afferent pathway may cause the bladder to be overactive. The afferent and efferent pathways to the bladder can be viewed as the lanes of a two-way street with impulses coming and going at all times. As the bladder stretches, nerves in the bladder wall and lining (urothelium) respond by sending messages (nerve impulses) to the brain via the afferent pathway through the spinal cord. These messages tell the brain that the bladder needs to contract. The brain then sends impulses back to the bladder along the **efferent pathway** telling it to contract.

Efferent pathway
the pathway that messages (nerve impulse signals) travel on between the central nervous system and the peripheral nervous system.

There is little information available about heredity and overactive bladder. In studies of twins, it appeared that OAB with urge incontinence might be hereditary. In children with OAB there is often a family member with OAB. In a recent study of urinary incontinence in women, there did appear to be a link between heredity and the development of urinary incontinence. The study found that for women whose mothers or older sisters were incontinent there was an increased risk for both stress and mixed (stress plus urge) incontinence, possibly with severe symptoms.

10. How common is overactive bladder?

Overactive bladder is very common. Previous studies estimated that about 16% of Americans suffer from overactive bladder and that worldwide between 50 and 100 million individuals suffer from it. Recent studies suggest that overactive bladder may be even more common. Overactive bladder affects both men and women, and the likelihood of having it increases with age. (See Figure 2.) Although OAB may develop at any time for both men and women, it tends to develop in men over the age of 60 years, whereas in women it tends to develop in the mid 40s. Urgency incontinence is more common in women than men. It occurs in 9.3% of women with OAB and in 2.6% of men with OAB.

Prevalence of OAB by Age

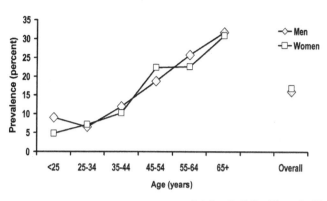

Data from the National Overactive BLadder
Evaluation (NOBLE) Research Program

Figure 2   Prevelance of overactive bladder as determined by the Noble study. *Source:* Stewart WF, VanRooyen JB, Cundiff GW, Abrams P, Herzog AR, Corey R, and Wein AJ. Prevalence and Burden of Overactive Bladder in the United States. *World J Urology* 20(6):327–36, 2003 May.

11. What is the natural history of overactive bladder? Is it permanent, can it go away, or does it come and go?

There is little information on the natural history of overactive bladder. The few studies that have been done suggest that OAB is a chronic, lifelong condition in adults that have it. In one study that followed patients with overactive bladder for as long as 10 years, bladder overactivity persisted in 69% of the patients, regardless of their treatment. Making changes to your diet and lifestyle may improve symptoms.

In children it appears that overactive bladder is a temporary condition that usually goes away on its own. There are no long-term studies, though, to determine whether these children develop symptoms again later in life.

12. How is overactive bladder diagnosed?

Your doctor will evaluate you in order to determine if your symptoms are due to OAB. The evaluation has two purposes: (1) to determine if your symptoms are related to OAB, and (2) to rule out other conditions that may cause or mimic OAB. (See Question 14.) Your doctor may have you fill out a bladder health questionnaire that will allow him or her to screen for possible bladder troubles. The following questions are often asked for screening purposes:

Over the past four weeks:

- Did you wake up at night to urinate two or more times?
- Did you have a sudden and uncomfortable feeling that you had to urinate soon?
- Were you bothered or concerned about bladder control?
- Did you lose or leak urine for any reason?
- Did you wear a pad or other material to absorb urine that you may have lost?

Symptom Assessment

A symptom assessment will focus on your urinary symptoms, such as how often you urinate, whether you have urgency, and if there is leakage. During this assessment, your doctor will try to determine whether your symptoms are related to OAB, stress incontinence, or a combination of the two (mixed urinary incontinence). Your doctor will probably ask whether straining, coughing, laughing, or sneezing causes leakage.

Optional Tools for Consideration: Bladder Diary

Day 1   Date: __/__/__   Number of pads used today:____

TIME	FLUIDS		URINATION					ACCIDENTS		
	What did you drink?	How much?	How many times?	How much each time? (S=small, M=moderate, L=large)	Did you have to rush to the bathroom?	Did you hurt yourself or fall down rushing to the bathroom?	What activity did it interrupt?	Did you have any accidents this time? (Sudden loss of urine)	How much urine did you leak? (S=small, M=moderate, L=large)	What were you doing at the time? (Exercising, sleeping, relaxing, etc.)
SAMPLE 12 PM	Juice	Tall glass	1	(S) M L	(Yes) No	Yes (No)	Walking the dog	(Yes) No	(S) M L	Gardening
				S M L	Yes No	Yes No		Yes No	S M L	
				S M L	Yes No	Yes No		Yes No	S M L	
				S M L	Yes No	Yes No		Yes No	S M L	
				S M L	Yes No	Yes No		Yes No	S M L	
				S M L	Yes No	Yes No		Yes No	S M L	
				S M L	Yes No	Yes No		Yes No	S M L	
				S M L	Yes No	Yes No		Yes No	S M L	
				S M L	Yes No	Yes No		Yes No	S M L	
				S M L	Yes No	Yes No		Yes No	S M L	
				S M L	Yes No	Yes No		Yes No	S M L	

Notes:_____   13

Figure 3   Simple bladder diary.

It is often helpful for you to fill out a bladder diary over several days to track your fluid intake and urinary symptoms. (See Figure 3.) In addition, your doctor will want to know if you are bothered by these symptoms. If you are not bothered, and you are not suffering from recurrent urinary tract or skin infections, there is no need to treat you. (For more information on voiding diaries, see Question 25.)

History and Physical Examination

A medical history, physical examination, and urinalysis are helpful in ruling out other conditions that mimic or cause OAB (see Question 14). When talking about your history, your doctor will want to know about your prior and current medical and surgical histories, what medications you are taking, including over-the-counter medications and herbal therapies, and if you have allergies. Questions about the medical status of your relatives may be asked. In addition, several questions about your diet and lifestyle will be asked. These may include: how much fluid you typically drink during the day, how much of that fluid is caffeinated, your occupation, and your ease of access to restrooms at work.

The physical exam will focus on your lower abdomen and perineum. Often a brief neurological evaluation will be included. The doctor will press on your lower abdomen to see if your bladder is distended. In women, a pelvic exam will determine if there is **pelvic prolapse**, a bulge visible in the vaginal area which may be related to propulse of the bowel, rectum, or uterus into the vagina. For women, during the examination of the perineum your doctor may ask you to strain, bear down, or cough to determine if there is any loss of control of urine. Your doctor may put a small cotton swab into the urethra and then ask you to strain; this is another method used to check for stress urinary incontinence. Your doctor may also perform an assessment of your pelvic floor muscle tone.

Pelvic prolapse

a weakening in the group of muscles that support the bladder, part of the urethra and in part of the female pelvic organ.

A rectal exam is often performed to check anal muscle tone. For men, the rectal examination includes a prostate examination to check the size of the prostate and to determine if there are nodules that may be a sign of prostate cancer.

Urinalysis

Urinalysis

a test that determines whether urine is normal or abnormal.

A **urinalysis** is a test to rule out a urinary tract infection. If the test shows that there are red blood cells in your urine, but you don't have a urinary tract infection, your doctor will need to determine if you have a bladder tumor or stone. If there are red blood cells in your urine you will also need to undergo a cystoscopy. A **cystoscopy** is an examination of the bladder and urethra through a narrow, telescope-like device that is passed through the urethra into the bladder. In addition, your doctor will check the results of your test for signs of diabetes, kidney disease, and the inability of the kidney to hold fluids back.

Additional Studies

Depending on your age, voiding symptoms, and medical and surgical history, you may need additional studies. In men who may have an obstruction from an enlarged prostate, and in elderly patients, patients with recurrent urinary tract infections, and those with neurological diseases, the doctor may perform a bladder scan after the individual has urinated to ensure that the bladder is emptying properly. Less commonly, a catheter may be passed through the urethra into the bladder to drain the bladder and then measure the amount of urine drained out. Your doctor may also perform a **bladder scan** by placing a small ultrasound probe on your lower abdomen after you urinate to determine if there is any urine left in the bladder. If there is urine left in the bladder, the probe will estimate the amount. Younger individuals should be able to completely empty their bladder. As you get older, though, there is likely a small amount of urine left in the bladder after urinating. More than 150 cc of urine left in the bladder after voiding could indicate either outlet obstruction or poor bladder contractibility.

If you have complex medical problems, if you have had prior bladder or urethral surgery, or if your earlier attempts at therapy for overactive bladder failed, your doctor may request that you undergo a urodynamic study (see Question 7).

Cystoscopy

a procedure in which the bladder and urethra are examined through a narrow telescope-like device that is passed through the urethra into the bladder.

Bladder scan

a simple ultrasound-like test which determines how much urine is in the bladder.

21

13. Is waking up at night caused by an overactive bladder?

Nocturia is defined as waking up one or more times at night to void. Nocturia is very common and appears to become more frequent as you get older. Nocturia is common with an overactive bladder, but there are several other important causes including:

- Cardiovascular disease, including congestive heart failure and circulatory problems
- Diabetes mellitus—elevated blood sugar
- Diabetes insipidus, which is a condition that is either related to a brain or kidney problem and results in the overproduction of urine
- Sleep apnea, which is a breathing problem that occurs during sleep
- Lower urinary tract obstruction such as that related to prostate enlargement
- Sleep problems
- Behavioral and environmental factors
- Nocturnal polyuria, which is when urine output during the day is normal, but at night is in excess of what is normal
- Polyuria, which is when the urine output for a 24-hr period is excessive

Bladder diary

a chart that a patient fills out to list the amount of urine they void and the number of times they void over a period of time.

To determine whether your nocturia is related to overactive bladder, your doctor will review your history and medications and ask you to fill out a **bladder diary**. (See Question 25.) This diary helps your physician to determine the potential cause of your nocturia. Treatment of your nocturia will vary with the cause. Studies have shown that if the cause of the nocturia is overactive bladder, antimuscarinics will help to decrease the number of times that you need to void at night.

14. Are there medical conditions that may cause or mimic overactive bladder?

There are several conditions that may cause symptoms typical of overactive bladder. Temporary or reversible conditions include:

1. urinary tract infection
2. estrogen deficiency in women
3. drug side effects (see Table 2)
4. excessive urine output
5. restricted mobility
6. severe constipation
7. altered mental status (see Table 3)

Other conditions that can contribute to, or may be associated with, overactive bladder include:

1. obstruction to the outflow of urine from the bladder
2. pelvic prolapse (descent of the bladder and other pelvic organs out of the pelvis)
3. significant stress incontinence

The acronym DIAPPERS can be used to describe potentially treatable causes of urinary incontinence:

- **Delirium** (confusion)
- **Infection**
- **Atrophic vaginitis** (low or absent estrogen levels before or after menopause, or after hysterectomy and oophorectomy [removal of the uterus and ovaries])

Atrophic vaginitis
a condition in which a woman has little or no estrogen before or after menopause, or after hysterectomy and oophorectomy (removal of the uterus and ovaries).

Table 2   Medications that may cause side effects that contribute to urinary incontinence

Drug Class	Side Effects
Alcohol	Polyuria, frequency, urgency, sedation, delirium
Alpha-agonists (e.g., pseudoephedrine, ephedrine)	Urinary retention
Alpha-blockers (e.g., tamsulosin (Flomax), doxazosin (Cardura), terazosin (Hytrin))	Urethral relaxation
ACE inhibitors, type I	Diuresis, cough with relaxation of pelvic floor
Anticholinergics (e.g., Oxybutynin (Ditropan), tolterodine (Detrol), solifenacin (Vesicare), trospium chloride (Sanctura), darifenacin (Enablex))	Urinary retention, overflow incontinence, stool impaction
Antidepressants (e.g., imipramine [Tofranil])	See anticholinergic side effects, sedation
Antiparkinsonism medications	Urinary urgency, constipation
Antipsychotics	See anticholinergic side effects, sedation, rigidity
Beta-agonists	Urinary retention
Caffeine	Bladder irritability that may aggravate or cause urge incontinence
Calcium-channel blockers	Urinary retention
Diuretics	Polyuria, urinary frequency, urgency
Sedatives/hypnotics	Sedation, delirium, immobility

Table 3 Management of conditions that cause reversible urinary incontinence

Condition	Management
Difficulty getting to or unwillingness to go to the toilet	
Delirium	Identification and management of the cause of the confused state of mind
Impaired mobility	Regular toileting, use of toilet substitutes (i.e., bedside commode, urinal)
Psychological problems	Appropriate psychological therapy
Drug side effects	If appropriate, discontinuation or decreased dosage of the drug, or changing to an alternative drug
Increased urine production	
Hyperglycemia	Improved control of blood sugars
Hypercalcemia	Treatment of the cause of the hypercalcemia
Excess fluid intake	Restriction of fluid intake and avoidance of caffeinated fluids
Fluid overload	
Venous insufficiency with lower extremity edema	Support hose (TEDs), elevation of legs, low sodium diet
Congestive heart failure	Medical therapy to optimize cardiac function
Urinary tract infection	Antibiotic therapy
Atrophic vaginitis/ urethritis	Topical estrogen therapy if not at risk for use of estrogen therapy
Stool impaction	Disimpaction (manual removal of stool), institution of therapy to prevent constipation including: increased fiber and fluids, stool softeners, and/or laxatives if needed

Diagnosis of Overactive Bladder

- **P**harmaceutical agents (medications)
- **P**sychologic (depression, dementia)
- **E**xcess urine output (secondary to increased fluid intake, increased renal production of urine, or over-flow incontinence)
- **R**estricted mobility (difficulty with ambulation—walking—related to musculoskeletal problems or environmental factors)
- **S**tool impaction (significant constipation)

15. Can men have prostate problems and overactive bladder or is it all just related to the prostate?

Lower urinary tract symptoms (LUTS) is a term used to describe two types of lower urinary tract symptoms: obstructive and irritative. Men with enlarged prostates often have obstructive symptoms such as a slow stream, hesitancy, intermittent stream, and straining; they may also experience dribbling after voiding.

Lower urinary tract symptoms

the term used to describe irritating voiding symptoms and/or symptoms due to obstruction.

About 40% to 60% of men with an enlarged prostate and bladder outlet obstruction have irritative symptoms. These include daytime frequency, nocturia, urgency, and sometimes urge incontinence. These symptoms suggest an overactive bladder. Up to 38% of men with benign prostate enlargement who have surgery for it still suffer from irritative symptoms afterward. This means they have two conditions: obstruction due to an enlarged prostate *and* overactive bladder. In some men, though, prostate surgery does improve their overactive bladder symptoms. Why this occurs is not fully understood. Some men may have overactive bladder only and no prostatic enlargement.

16. What is the impact of overactive bladder?

Overactive bladder clearly has a negative effect on quality of life. Studies have shown that urge incontinence has more of a negative effect on quality of life than stress incontinence. This makes sense, because with stress incontinence you have an element of control. If you avoid coughing, laughing, sneezing, or exertion, you can avoid leaking. With urge incontinence, though, there is no warning or control.

Overactive bladder and urinary incontinence may affect quality of life in a variety of ways:

- Psychological—it may lead to guilt/depression, loss of self-esteem, fear of being a burden, and fear of lack of bladder control that will lead to the smell of urine.
- Social—you may avoid going out socially, or may plan outings around toilet accessibility.
- Domestic—there is a need for specialized pads and protective underwear; for some this may create a financial burden. Also, the elderly may have to rely on a caregiver to obtain these items.
- Occupational—may lead to absences from work, decreased productivity, and difficulties with colleagues at work.
- Sexual—may lead to avoidance of sexual activity and intimacy.
- Physical—may lead to limitation or a complete stop of physical activity, particularly for those who suffer from mixed incontinence.

Studies have shown that about 50% of nursing home patients are admitted because of urinary incontinence. In the elderly, urinary incontinence is associated with an increased risk of urinary tract infections, skin infections, and irritation. In older women, having an overactive bladder and urinary incontinence is related to a rise in the risk of falls and bone fractures.

17. Is overactive bladder treatable?

Yes. Most people will notice significant improvement in their symptoms when they *combine* behavioral modification and medical therapy (see Questions 24–28). People who do not improve with this combined approach, or who are unable to use this approach for medical reasons, may be treated in a different way, such as with intravesical capsaicin or resiniferatoxin, or sacral neuromodulation (see Questions 29 and 34–38). On rare occasions these approaches don't work. If this is the case, your doctor may try:

1. injecting your bladder with botulinum toxin;
2. procedures to make your bladder larger; or
3. **bladder denervation** procedures, which interrupt the nerves and prevent the bladder muscle from being stimulated to contract. (See Questions 30–33 and 40–43.)

Bladder denervation

procedures that deaden or eliminate the nerves in the urethra, bladder, or rectum in an effort to interrupt the nerve supply to the bladder and stop bladder contractions.

When you discuss treatment options with your doctor it is essential that you talk about expectations. For example, if you currently void 20 times and have 6 incontinent episodes a day, it may not be realistic to expect to be dry all the time and void only 6 times a day. A reasonable expectation may be to cut your current number of voiding and incontinence episodes by half.

18. Is overactive bladder curable?

A combination of medical therapy and behavioral modification improves overactive bladder symptoms in up to 85% of people. In addition, it is important to remember that in most cases, medical therapy does not lead to any permanent or long-lasting changes. So, if you are doing well on medical therapy and suddenly stop the therapy, the likelihood is that your overactive bladder symptoms will return.

PART THREE

Treatment of Overactive Bladder

What are the options for treating overactive bladder?

What are Kegel (pelvic floor muscle) exercises?

What is neuromodulation/sacral nerve stimulation?

More . . .

19. What are the options for treating overactive bladder?

Several treatments are available. Some are not invasive, such as behavioral therapy and oral medication. Invasive approaches include placing medication directly in your bladder (**intravesically**) and surgery. Typically, you begin with behavioral therapy and oral medications. If these don't work, you will move on to intravesical and surgical therapies.

First-line treatments for the management of overactive bladder include:

- Behavioral therapy (see Figure 4)
- Medications

Second-line treatments include:

- Intravesical therapy (capsaicin and resiniferatoxin—see Question 29)
- Injection of botulinum toxin into the bladder (see Questions 30–33)

Intravesical

medication placed directly into the bladder.

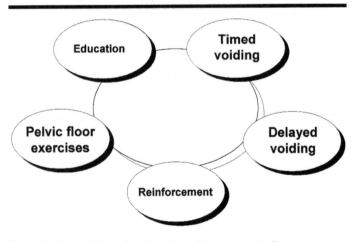

Behavioral Modification

Education

Timed voiding

Pelvic floor exercises

Delayed voiding

Reinforcement

Figure 4   Types of behavioral therapy and management of symptoms.

- Sacral neuromodulation (electrical stimulatio—see Questions 34–39)

Third-line treatments include:

- Bladder augmentation (see Questions 40–42)
- Urinary diversion (a procedure designed to bypass the bladder)
- Bladder denervation procedures (see Question 43)

NONINVASIVE OPTIONS

20. What medications are available to treat overactive bladder? Is there anyone who should not take an antimuscarinic medication?

Several medications are available. Their goal is to prevent or at least decrease the number of uninhibited bladder contractions, which will lead to less urinary frequency, urgency, and urge incontinence. Currently, **antimuscarinic** medications are the gold standard for management of overactive bladder. Antimuscarinics have been shown to increase bladder capacity and prevent uninhibited bladder contractions; however, their use has been limited in the past due to a high incidence of side effects. OAB can make even basic tasks of daily life challenging. It is important to have drugs that treat symptoms of OAB without causing negative side effects. Thus one of the main goals for creating new drugs is to decrease the side effects of the drugs that exist. As part of this process, researchers have explored many ways for people to take these drugs, to try and improve the side effects. Such changes include:

1. Taking a long-acting pill once a day

Antimuscarinic agents

a type of medication that produces effects that block the muscarinic receptor, which is involved in the control of bladder muscle contraction.

Transdermal

medication is delivered to the body by a skin patch.

2. Absorbing the drug through a skin patch (**transdermally**)

3. Having the drug placed directly in the bladder (intravesically)

Individuals with urinary retention, certain stomach problems, narrow angle glaucoma, or anyone at risk of developing any one of these conditions should not use antimuscarinics. If you have glaucoma, the safest thing to do is to check with your eye doctor before taking an antimuscarinic. You should also talk to your doctor before taking antimuscarinics if you have liver or kidney failure. Question 23 discusses the side effects of antimuscarinics.

21. How do antimuscarinics decrease overactive bladder symptoms?

As described in Question 1, a neurotransmitter called acetylcholine binds with muscarinic receptors in the bladder. This causes the bladder to contract. Antimuscarinics prevent acetylcholine from binding to the receptors in the bladder, so the bladder has less involuntary contractions. Antimuscarinics work fairly quickly; within one to two weeks you should notice improvement. It may take up to 3 months before the drug's full potential is reached. As antimuscarines prevent involuntary contractions, they should not prevent you from urinating when you want to.

22. How long should I expect to take my anitmuscarinic medication?

In terms of determining if the medication is going to help you or not you will know pretty quickly, within a week or so, however, it may take up to 3 months for the full benefits of the medication to be seen so continue with the medicaton for at least a month to see if it is working as well as you and your doctor would like. Remember, that overactive bladder is a "chronic" condition in most adults, which means that you will most likely have an overactive bladder for the long-term. The antimuscarinic medication controls your bladder only when you are taking the medication which means that if you want to continue controlling your bladder you will need to continue taking the medication for the long-term. There are a few individuals, who are able to stop the antimuscarinic medications after a while but most people will need to stay on the medications if they wish to control their overactive bladder symptoms.

23. What are the available antimuscarinics and what are their side effects?

The following antimuscarinics are used in the United States:

1. Detrol LA (Pfizer)
2. oxybutynin (generic)
3. Ditropan XL (Johnson & Johnson)
4. transdermal oxybutynin (Oxytrol) (Watson)

Other approved medications are:

1. trospium chloride (Sanctura, Indevus)
2. solifenacin (Vesicare, Astellas)
3. darifenacin (Enablex, Novartis)

All of these medications are effective. Because they each are a little different, your doctor will work with you to ensure that the best drug for you is chosen to treat your symptoms. A brief description of how each drug works, how it is taken, and its side effects, follows.

Detrol LA

Tolterodine is an antimuscarinic. Detrol is a pill taken twice a day. Detrol LA is a long-acting version taken once a day. Although tolterodine is an antimuscarinic, it has a lower incidence of dry mouth and constipation than oxybutynin. By taking the medication at night you can have even a lower risk of dry mouth and constipation. Detrol has been shown to be helpful in a variety of people with OAB including: elderly patients, males, and patients with severe urinary incontinence. Detrol is the world's number-one prescribed medication for overactive bladder. It is the most widely researched drug for this condition, supported by more data than any other OAB medication.

Oxybutynin (generic)

Oxybutynin is an antimuscarinic that has been used for a long time and is now manufactured by several generic companies. It can be taken up to four times a day, or crushed and dissolved in sterile water, and given through a catheter inserted in the bladder. It has a high likelihood of causing dry mouth and constipation.

Ditropan XL

This is the long-acting form of oxybutynin and is taken once a day. (The capsule itself does not break down, so don't be alarmed if you see it floating in the toilet bowl or in your colostomy bag if you have a bowel bag!) This capsule can't be crushed or cut, as it will no longer be 'long acting.' The side effects of Ditropan XL are the same as for oxybutynin and other antimuscarinics: dry mouth and constipation, but they tend to be less frequent and less bothersome than oxybutynin.

Oxtrol (transdermal oxybutynin)

Transdermal oxybutynin (Watson) is absorbed through a skin patch. The patch can be worn on the abdomen, buttock, or hip. A new site should be used for each new patch to avoid using the same place twice within a seven-day period. The patch is left on for about three days at a time and then changed. The side effects are dry mouth and constipation but much lower than oxybutynin and Ditropan XL. Some people may develop redness and itching at the site where the patch is placed. This symptom may be worse for the elderly, who have thin, sensitive skin.

Santura (trospium chloride)

Trospium chloride (Indevus) is an antimuscarinic that was recently approved for use in the United States. It is usually taken twice a day and should not be taken within one hour of eating. An advantage of this medication is that it has little reaction with other medications. Trospium chloride also causes dry mouth and constipation.

Vesicare (solifenacin)

Solifenacin (Astellas) is another antimuscarinic, which recently was approved by the FDA for use in the United States. It is taken as a pill once a day, and, as for other antimuscarinics, dry mouth and constipation are side effects. The pill can't be crushed or cut. It is available in two doses.

Enablex (darifenacin)

Darifenacin (Novartis) is an antimuscarinic that was recently approved for use in the United States. It is taken as a pill once a day, and its side effects are dry mouth and constipation. The tablet cannot be crushed or cut. It is available in two doses.

Less commonly used medications

Propantheline bromide (generic). Pro-banthine is also an antimuscarinic. It is a pill that usually is taken four times a day. However, each person that takes it may need a different dose. Its side effects are dry mouth and constipation.

Probantheline bromide

A nonselective antimuscarinic medication for overactive bladder; individual doses will vary.

Antidepressants

Imipramine (generic) is an antidepressant that acts like an antimuscarinic. It is taken as a pill; the dose varies. Imipramine can have serious side effects on the cardiovascular system, including lowering blood pressure when you go from a sitting to standing position and abnormal heart rhythms. Because of this, it should be kept out of the reach of young children. If you decide to stop taking imipramine after being on it for a long time, it is important to do so under your doctor's supervision as opposed to stopping it suddenly.

Imipramine

an antidepressant medication that is occasionally used for overactive bladder; it has antimuscarinic properties and acts on two neurotransmitters in the brain (sertotonin and noradrenaline) involved in the complex interactions related to normal bladder filling and emptying.

How to minimize side effects

The following is a list of side effects and how you can minimize them.

- Dry mouth—The saliva your mouth makes when you're not eating coats your teeth and gums and maintains the health of your mouth. Frequent sips of water, drinking milk, use of olive oil to moisten your mouth, and sugar-free gum and other sugar-free candies help stimulate your salivary glands. Avoid drinks with caffeine or alcohol and avoid smoking. Using an antiseptic mouthwash is helpful for keeping your mouth clean and reducing the amount of bacteria in it. Glycerin and lemon mouthwashs can be used to try and stimulate saliva production. However, these should be used sparingly because overuse can cause tooth decay and gum disease. Use of high concentration fluoride toothpastes can also help prevent cavities.

- Constipation—To minimize the effects of constipation make sure you drink enough fluids, increase your fiber intake, and use stool softeners and stimulants/laxatives as needed. If you are prone to constipation, it is very helpful to get your bowels regular before you begin taking antimuscarinics. Some medications have a higher risk of constipation than others so if you have a problem with constipation talk to your doctor to make sure that you are put on an OAB medication that is less likely to cause constipation.

- Central nervous system—Several antimuscarinics have side effects that affect the central nervous system. Central nervous system side effects include headache, dizziness, and sleepiness. Some medications, like oxybutynin, may affect **cognition** (thinking, learning, and memory) in certain people. Medications such as tolterodine, trospium, and darifenacin are less likely to have these side effects. Your doctor will discuss these issues with you when deciding what medication you should take.

Cognition
general term encompassing thinking, learning, and memory.

- Urinary retention—In rare cases, antimuscarinics cause **urinary retention**, leaving the patient unable

Urinary retention
the inability to urinate.

to urinate. In most cases, the patient will be able to void again after your bladder recovers. Your doctor will discuss this possible side effect with you.

24. What is behavioral therapy and what is its success rate? Can I combine an antimuscarinic drug with behavioral therapy?

Behavioral therapy
a group of treatments designed for educating an individual about his/her medical condition so strategies can be developed to minimize or eliminate the symptoms.

Behavioral therapy is often the first approach used to treat overactive bladder. Studies show that combining behavioral therapy with medication works better than using medication alone. Behavioral therapy focuses on understanding your bladder, its condition, and your pelvic floor muscles. Its goals are to reduce or eliminate incontinence episodes and urinary frequency.

There are several parts to behavioral therapy, starting with patient education. (See Figure 4.) Your doctor will explain to you the basics of how the bladder, urethra, and pelvic muscles function as well as the role of the bladder and the pelvic floor muscles in voiding and staying dry. Behavioral therapy includes keeping a voiding diary, making changes in your diet, practicing timed voiding, and doing pelvic floor (Kegel) muscle exercises. These are described in Question 27.

Success rate

Compliance
the consistency and accuracy with which a patient follows the regimen prescribed by a physician or other healthcare professional.

Behavioral therapy works but requires motivation and **compliance**. You must do the exercises and make the changes to your diet and lifestyle as your doctors prescribe. It may feel like a lot of work, but the benefits are real. For the elderly, there is often the added need of a dedicated caregiver to assist with behavioral therapy.

You can most definitely combine an antimuscarinic medication with behavioral therapy. In fact, studies have shown that a combination of the two gives the best results. I usually recommend that my patients do both, realizing that the medical therapy is going to provide the "quick fix" but that the behavioral therapy, although it takes a bit longer, will add to the improvement in your symptoms. You can start the two of the therapies together or you can start with one of the two therapies and add the second one if you wish to improve your symptoms further.

25. What is a bladder diary?

A bladder diary (see Figure 3, in Question 12) is used to help the patient and physician understand the patient's lower urinary tract function. Typically, your doctor will ask you to fill out a daily voiding diary for several days to see your voiding pattern. The diary also is helpful in the future for evaluating your response to treatment.

The bladder diary has several parts. One section is for the amount you void and the time of each void. You'll also record the number and severity of incontinence episodes and when they occur the degree of urgency and pad usage. The volume and type of fluid you drink are also recorded. This allows for identification of those individuals who drink excessive amounts of fluid or who have a high intake of caffeinated fluids.

Caffeine is a diuretic; it makes the kidneys produce increased amounts of urine). It is also a bladder irritant. Those with high fluid intake (more than 2.5 quart per day) may benefit from reducing it. Highly acidic diets or overzealous intake of cranberry products, juice, or pills, may lead to acidic urine, which also may irritate the bladder. Lastly, not drinking enough can make the urine concentrated, and this too may irritate the bladder. When you are drinking an appropriate amount of fluids for your bodily needs, your urine should be light yellow.

26. What is timed voiding?

Timed voiding
a type of therapy that involves urinating at two- to three-hour intervals, no matter if there is an urge.

Timed voiding is an important part of behavioral therapy. Typically, you are asked to void, whether you feel the urge or not, every two to three hours. (If you suffer from urinary frequency you may already be voiding more frequently than this.) For those who suffer from urge incontinence, timed voiding ensures regular emptying of the bladder and should decrease the volume of urine that you leak during an urge incontinent episode. In the elderly, a caregiver will be required to prompt voiding and help the person get to and from the bathroom.

If you suffer from urgency and frequency without urge incontinence, you can try to delay voiding. With delayed voiding, you consciously try to ignore the urge sensation and hold your urine for a progressively longer period of time to gradually increase the amount of fluid your bladder can hold. This technique will be easier if your urine is less irritating to your bladder.

27. What are pelvic floor muscle (Kegel) exercises?

Pelvic floor muscles
a group of muscles that form a sling or hammock across the opening of the pelvis; these muscles, together with their surrounding tissue, are responsible for keeping all of the pelvic organs (bladder, uterus, and rectum) in place and functioning correctly.

If you have urge incontinence, there is a problem with your bladder and your **pelvic floor muscles**. Pelvic floor muscles are a group of muscles that are attached to the pelvic bone and act like a hammock to support the pelvic organs, which include the bladder, uterus, and rectum. These muscles may be weakened by childbirth, prior pelvic surgery, or obesity. Contracting, or tightening, pelvic floor muscles appears to prevent bladder contractions. In 1948 Dr. Arnold Kegel developed pelvic floor muscle exercises for stress incontinence, but they are helpful for OAB as well. They have a cure rate of up to 84%.

As mentioned in Question 24, you must do Kegel exercises on a regular basis in order for them to work. Similar to weight lifting, strengthening the pelvic floor muscles requires repeated contractions on a daily basis. If you don't stick to a regular schedule, the exercises won't work.

People may find it hard to identify the pelvic floor muscles and contract them. Typically, when someone is asked to contract their pelvic floor muscles, the buttocks are tightened. Actually, neither the buttock nor the thigh muscles are involved in these exercises. Placing a finger or special weight (called a vaginal cone) in the vagina (for women) or anus (for men) and contracting the pelvic floor muscles produces a tightening around the finger, or keep the weight from falling out if a woman is in a standing position. If you have a difficult time identifying your pelvic floor muscles, biofeedback can be used (see Question 28). Some individuals may experience some muscle discomfort or feelings of sexual arousal after starting a pelvic floor muscle exercise program.

A good way to start Kegel exercises is to perform them for five minutes twice a day. You should tighten/squeeze the pelvic floor muscles for a count of 4, and then relax for a count of 4, and repeat this for a total of five minutes. If you can't do this for a full five minutes at the start, start with a tolerable time and gradually build up to five minutes. The exercises can be done anytime and anywhere. It is easiest to perform the exercises at the same times each day to help build a routine.

Who is a candidate for them?

Kathy's comment:

Almost anyone is a candidate for Kegel exercises. This is especially true if you leak urine. My experience is a little bit out of the ordinary. As a nurse, I have taught patients how to do Kegel exercises, which allowed me to use the technique efficiently as soon as I started. Nevertheless, it was clear to me early on that you have to be very dedicated and extremely motivated to achieve success. Finally, it is important to realize that these exercises are for the long term. As with any muscle group, if you stop exercising them they will weaken.

The ideal candidate for Kegel exercises is highly motivated. Because Kegel exercises help with stress, urge, and mixed urinary incontinence, everyone is a candidate for them.

How successful are they?

Kathy's comment:

I tried Kegel exercises without success for stress incontinence. However, I was having some urge incontinence. I did notice an improvement with the urge incontinence, but it took a few months, just like it takes to strengthen other muscles.

You will not notice results right away. It takes time to strengthen the pelvic floor muscles and they will only remain strong when you do the exercises on a regular basis. In most women, it will take 6 to 12 weeks to notice a change in urine loss, provided that the exercises are being performed properly and regularly. At the earliest, men will notice results a month after beginning the exercises.

28. What is biofeedback?

Biofeedback is information you can get about your body's normally unconscious processes. You become aware of this information through visual (see), auditory (hear), or tactile (touch) signals.

An **electromyography** is used to evaluate pelvic floor muscle activity. It measures the activity of certain muscles by using electrodes that are placed near or into the muscles. To evaluate the pelvic floor muscles, the electrodes may be placed on the skin near the anus, or special probes may be placed into the vagina, anus, or urethra. These electrodes are connected to a machine that shows the activity of the muscles on a screen and records it onto a paper tracing. Relaxation of the pelvic floor muscles makes a flat line on the tracing; contraction of the muscles causes an up-and-down line on the tracing. By watching the screen you will be able to tell when you are relaxing or contracting your pelvic floor muscles.

Who is a candidate?

Not everyone needs biofeedback. You are a candidate for biofeedback if you are having trouble identifying your pelvic floor muscles, or if your pelvic floor muscle exercises aren't working after you've been doing them for some time.

What is the success rate?

The combination of behavioral therapy (dietary and lifestyle changes, voiding regiments), including Kegel exercises, and biofeedback, works better than behavioral therapy alone. However, biofeedback works better for stress urinary incontinence than for urge incontinence. Younger women and those without estrogen deficiency

Biofeedback
information about one or more of an individual's normally unconscious body processes is made available to the individual through a visual (see), auditory (hear), or tactile (touch) signal.

Electromyography
type of noninvasive test using skin patches to measure the activity in muscles.

tend to do better with biofeedback than older women and women with low estrogen levels.

29. What are capsaicin and resiniferatoxin?

Capsaicin

the active ingredient found in chili peppers used to decrease bladder overactivity.

Resiniferatoxin

a chemical derived from a cactus-like plant, Euphorbia resinifera, that can decrease bladder overactivity.

Capsaicin is the active ingredient found in chili peppers. **Resiniferatoxin** is a chemical derived from a cactus-like plant, *Euphorbia resinifera*. Both of these are much hotter than the hottest pepper.

How do they work?

There are two types of nerves inside the bladder that travel from the bladder to the central nervous system. These nerves are responsible for transmitting signals of bladder fullness and/or bladder discomfort from the bladder to the brain. One type of nerve, called the small A delta fiber, sends signals about bladder fullness. The second type of nerve, the C fiber, sends signals when the bladder is irritated or has pain.

When placed into the bladder, both capsaicin and resiniferatoxin cause an intense stimulation of the C fibers. This causes these bladder nerves to run out of neurotransmitters, so that there are less signals to the brain that would cause the bladder to contract. If you respond well to treatment with capsaicin or resiniferatoxin your results will last for several months.

Having capsaicin placed directly in the bladder is extremely uncomfortable. In fact, it is far too uncomfortable to be done without general or spinal anesthesia. Resiniferatoxin is actually stronger than capsaicin, but it does not require anesthesia because there is no intense pain when it is placed into the bladder.

How effective are they? How are they administered and how long will the response last?

Capsaicin helps decrease bladder overactivity. Studies have shown that it is more effective in people with overactive bladder from a neurogenic cause, such as from a spinal cord injury, multiple sclerosis, or myelomeningocele. It is less effective in people with overactive bladder symptoms from a nonneurologic cause—those with hypersensitive bladder and those with pelvic pain. Capsaicin may not work right away. In fact, it may be as long as two months before you notice any improvement. Some people may find that their symptoms get worse for one to two weeks before the symptoms disappear. If capsaicin does work for you, you'll find that the improvement lasts anywhere from three to six months to over a year.

Resiniferatoxin has been shown to improve OAB symptoms in people with overactive bladder from both neurologic and nonneurologic causes. In most cases, improvement starts as soon as one day after the treatment and lasts for at least three months.

What are the side effects?

As mentioned above, your symptoms may get worse temporarily for a week or two before they get better. Other possible side effects are pain above the pubic bone and around the perineum, burning sensation, urinary frequency, urinary incontinence, and hematuria (presence of red blood cells in the urine). Urinary tract infections can occur as a result of **catheterization** with either capsaicin or resiniferatoxin use. If the capsaicin

Catheterization
a tubular instrument especially designed to be passed through the urethra into the bladder to drain it of retained urine.

or resiniferatoxin leaks onto your skin, it may cause local skin irritation.

For people with a spinal cord injury and a condition called autonomic dysreflexia, there is a risk that capsaicin or resiniferatoxin might cause **hypertension** (a rise in blood pressure). In this case, the procedure should be done under anesthesia with continuous blood pressure monitoring. After the procedure, the person should be monitored closely and have a Foley catheter.

Hypertension

transitory or sustained elevated arterial blood pressure.

MINIMALLY INVASIVE OPTIONS

30. What is botulinum toxin?

Botulinum neurotoxin is one of the most poisonous biological chemicals known. It works by weakening and reducing activity in affected muscles and when injected into a specified muscle group, it can lead to paralysis of that muscle group. It does not spread to surrounding muscles.

Botulinum neurotoxin

a poisonous biological chemical produced by the bacterium Clostridium botulinum that is used medically to cause temporary muscle paralysis.

31. How does botulinum toxin work in overactive bladder?

Botulinum toxin prevents the release of the neurotransmitter acetylcholine. In the case of an overactive bladder, it is the release of acetylcholine that causes the bladder muscle to contract involutarily. When the release of acetylcholine is prevented, the bladder doesn't contract as much.

For the toxin to be effective it must be injected directly into the bladder muscle. This is done through the **cystoscope,** which is used for a procedure called a **cystoscopy.** The cystoscope, a long telescope-like instrument, is passed through the urethra into the

Cystoscope

a long telescope-like instrument that is passed through the urethra into the bladder to identify and treat urologic problems.

Cystoscopy

a procedure in which the bladder and urethra are examined through a cystoscope that is passed through the urethra into the bladder.

bladder. After the doctor inspects your bladder, the bladder muscle is injected with the botulinum toxin through a slender hollow needle that is passed through the cystoscope into the wall of the bladder. Because the toxin only works locally, about 30 to 40 injections of an extremely small amount of the toxin are used during the procedure.

32. How effective is botulinum toxin in overactive bladder?

For most people with overactive bladder, injections of botulinum toxin last for about three months. Therefore, the procedure must be repeated as needed.

Botulinum toxin bladder injection can also be used for people with overactive bladder as a result of spinal cord injury. The majority of these people experienced fewer incontinence episodes and the procedure appears to last for them for at least nine months.

33. What are the side effects of botulinum toxin?

In general, botulinum toxin doesn't have many side effects. In cases when the injection goes beyond the bladder wall, there may be an effect on muscles and tissue outside of the bladder.

Rarely, the injection is associated with a flu-like illness.

Botulinum toxin should not be used in pregnant women or women who are breastfeeding. The effects in children are not well known. The cystoscopy itself and injections may cause temporary irritation to the urethra and bladder, leading to short-term discomfort with urination (dysuria) and blood in the urine (hematuria). In rare cases you can develop a urinary tract infection. The long-term effects of botulinum toxin on the bladder muscle are not well known.

34. What is sacral neuromodulation (sacral nerve stimulation)?

Neuromodulation

surgical placement of a permanent continuous nerve stimulator and its electrode wires.

Neuromodulation is the process of electrically stimulating specific nerves (the sacral nerves) in the pelvis. It is thought that the "stimulated" nerves reduce the spastic activity of the pelvic floor muscles and improve the function of the urethral sphincter muscle. It is also thought that stimulation of certain other nerves, including sensory nerves, in the pelvic floor may prevent them from stimulating the bladder to contract.

35. Who is a candidate for sacral neuromodulation?

If medicine and behavioral therapy haven't worked for you, you are a candidate for sacral neuromodulation. Your doctor may consider sacral neuromodulation for you before considering invasive surgical procedures such as urinary diversion and bladder augmentation.

Sacrum

refers to the large, irregular, triangular-shaped bone made up of the five fused vertebrae below the lumbar region; comprises the pelvis.

Before having sacral neuromodulation you doctor will recommend a complete urologic and neurologic evaluation. This evaluation should include: a history; physical examination; urinalysis; radiologic evaluation of the kidneys, bladder, and lower spinal column including the **sacrum**; a urodynamic study; and a cystoscopy. This extensive evaluation is to ensure that there are no other conditions present that may cause or mimic the overactive bladder symptoms.

36. How is sacral neuromodulation performed?

You begin with a three- to four-day trial with a temporary neuromodulation device implanted in your abdomen. There are three steps for implanting the device:

1. Your doctor will identify the exact location of your sacral nerves.
2. External wires will be placed into the area in your pelvis where the nerves are located to determine your response to the electrical stimulation.
3. The device will be implanted.

A description of each of these steps follows.

Phase 1

This phase may be performed while you are under local or general anesthesia. While you are lying face down, your doctor applies pressure with his or her hands to your lower back to determine where the wires should be placed. Two needle electrodes, one on each side, are then placed into this area. Next your doctor will stimulate the electrodes to confirm that they are properly positioned. If the electrodes are in the proper positions, your pelvic floor muscles will contract with stimulation and your big toes will bend. If the needle electrodes are not in the correct position, your doctor will reposition them until they are in the right place.

Phase 2

Once the correct positions of the needle electrodes are confirmed, external stimulation wires replace them. These wires may be taped in place or tunneled under the skin to prevent them from falling out over the following three- to four-day test period. The external wires are connected to a portable hand-held neurostimulator. You will be sent home the same day and be asked to fill out a voiding diary over the next three to four days. On or before the fourth day you will undergo a urodynamic study (see Question 7) to assess your response to the device. A positive response is an improvement in your symptoms of at least 50%. At the end of the test the wires are removed.

Phase 3

If you responded well to the trial, you are a candidate for placement of the permanent device. Typically, there is at least a two-week period between the trial and placement of the permanent device to decrease your chance of developing an infection. The procedure for placing the permanent device is performed under general anesthesia. One, or more commonly, two (one on each side) permanent electrodes are placed into the area in the pelvis and are secured in place. The wires are then tunneled under the skin to bring them to the stimulating device, which is placed under the skin in the lower abdominal area.

37. What is the success rate of sacral neuromodulation?

Sacral neuromodulation only works in about 50% of people with urge incontinence. For those who test well and undergo permanent placement, about 60% have positive results for at least five years.

38. What are the risks of placement of a sacral neuromodulation device?

Overall, the complication rate is 22%–43% with a reoperation rate of 6%–50%. Complications may be related to the procedure or to the function of the device.

Surgical complications include:

- Discomfort related to the placement of the device and the tunneling of the electrode wires.
- Wound infections and infections around the neurostimulator device.
- Movement of the electrodes from their original sites.

Complications related to the device include:

- Uncomfortable sensations related to too much electrical current.
- Broken electrodes.
- Mechanical problems with the device.
- Battery exhaustion.

39. Are there other forms of electrical stimulation besides sacral nerve stimulation?

Yes, there are other forms of electrical stimulation that have been used to treat a variety of bladder conditions. Pelvic floor electrostimulation has been used to strengthen the sphincter, the muscles around the urethra, and the pelvic floor muscles. The devices for these forms of stimulation may be placed on the skin (**transcutaneous**) in the appropriate area. Electrical stimulation has been shown to increase bladder capacity. It has also been used for stress urinary incontinence.

Transcutaneous denotes the passage of substances through the unbroken skin.

53

SURGICAL OPTIONS

40. What is bladder augmentation?

Bladder augmentation is a surgical procedure for enlarging the bladder. Bladder size can be increased by adding other tissues to it, such as a part of your intestine or stomach, or a segment of ureter that has been dilated (made much wider than normal). (See Figure 4.) The bladder may also be enlarged by removing the detrusor muscle from the its lining (the mucosa). The goals of bladder augmentation are to:

- Enable storage of urine at a low bladder pressure.
- Help you to achieve continence.
- Avoid damage to your kidneys by keeping bladder pressure low.
- Allow you to empty your bladder in a timely and convenient manner.

41. Who is a candidate for bladder augmentation?

Bladder augmentation is an option for people for whom all other methods of treatment have failed. Those individuals with small bladder capacities, with elevated bladder pressures, and uninhibited bladder contractions with normal urethral sphincter function are the best candidates for bladder augmentation. It is essential that you discuss with your doctor the permanent nature of this procedure and the risks of each type of bladder augmentation.

Often, the bladder can't fully contract after augmentation. Because of this, if you are considering bladder augmentation you must be willing to take the risk that you will be dependent on **clean intermittent catheterization** (CIC) to empty your bladder for the rest of

Bladder augmentation

a surgical procedure whereby the bladder is enlarged.

Clean intermittent catheterization

a type of temporary catheter to remove urine from the body; usually self-accomplished by inserting the tube through the urethra to empty the bladder several times per day.

your life. To do this procedure you must first learn your own urological anatomy. You also must be able to reach the urethra and learn how to manipulate the catheter (tube) to empty your bladder properly. This is not difficult for most people after proper instruction.

42. What are the types of bladder augmentation?

There are several different ways to enlarge the bladder, including enterocystoplasty, gastrocystoplasty, auto-augmentation, and ureterocystoplasty.

Enterocystoplasty—Enterocystoplasty is the most common method for bladder augmentation. The surgery is performed under general anesthesia. Typically, it is performed through a midline abdominal cut (**incision**); however, some urologists are performing all or part of the procedure **laparoscopically**.

With enterocystoplasty, the bladder is made larger by the addition of a segment of small or large intestine. Traditionally, the ileum, which is a section of the small intestine, is used. The piece of intestine is removed and the remainder of the intestine is reconnected. The piece of intestine is then opened and made into a patch that is sewn to the bladder. Typically, a drainage tube, called a Foley catheter or a suprapubic tube, is left in place for at least a week to allow for healing. The hospital stay is usually around five to seven days, depending on when bowel function returns. A **cystogram**—a study in which fluid is inserted through the drainage tube into the bladder and x-rays are taken—is done to make sure closure between bowel and bladder is "water-tight" before the tube is removed. This procedure is successful in 77% of patients with OAB who haven't responded to other treatments.

Enterocystoplasty
a surgical procedure to enlarge the bladder by the addition of a segment of small or large intestine.

Incision
a cut; a surgical wound.

Laparoscopic
type of microsurgery using a tiny telescope, laparoscope passed through the skin and into the organ, with a fiberoptic camera and surgical tools inserted to view and perform the surgery.

Cystogram
a type of test where fluid called contrast material is inserted through the drainage tube placed into the bladder and x-rays are obtained. The contrast material causes specific areas of the body to be "lit up" by the x-rays so that the radiologist can see the area.

Disadvantages of the procedure include:

- Inability to urinate on your own after.
- Bleeding, infection, urinary leakage, and poor healing.
- As intra-abdominal scarring that can lead to bowel obstruction, urinary tract infections, bladder and kidney stones, and bladder rupture.
- The intestine continues to make mucus. Mucus can plug the catheter and increase the risk of stones and infections so you may need to wash the mucus out of your bladder (irrigate).
- There is a rare risk of cancer many years after the augmentation. After 5 years, your doctor will start checking your urine and performing cystoscopies to check for cancer.
- Even though the segment of intestine used for augmentation is sewn to the bladder, it still functions as if part of the intestine. Because of this, periodic blood testing is required. Some people will require medications to counteract the acid that is reabsorbed by the intestinal segment. In addition, electrolyte levels are often abnormal after enterocystoplasty, and need to be monitored.

Gastrocystoplasty

Gastrocystoplasty
similar to enterocystoplasty, except that instead of using a piece of intestine, a segment of the stomach is used to patch the bladder.

Gastrocystoplasty—Gastrocystoplasty is similar to enterocystoplasty, except that instead of using a piece of intestine, a piece of the stomach is used. This procedure is most commonly used in children with overactive bladder due to a neurologic abnormality.

Autoaugmentation
a surgical procedure in which a part of the bladder muscle—the detrusor—is removed from the bladder mucosa.

Autoaugmentation—Autoaugmentation is the surgical procedure in which a part of the bladder muscle, the detrusor, is removed from the bladder. When the muscle is removed from a part of the bladder, that part of the bladder is no longer able to contract. Since the procedure requires access only to the bladder, the surgery does not require entry into the abdominal cavity, only into the pelvis. This is a less invasive procedure and has a faster recovery, but it often doesn't work as well as enterocystoplasty.

Complications of autoaugmentation include:

- Lack of consistent improvement in bladder capacity.
- May require clean intermittent catheterization for bladder emptying (see Question 41).

Ureterocystoplasty—Ureterocystoplasty is a technique used in patients who have a dilated distal ureter, which can be isolated, opened, and used as a bladder patch. Only select people are candidates for this procedure.

Ureterocystoplasty

a technique used in patients who have a dilated distal ureter, which can be isolated, opened, and used as a bladder patch.

43. What are bladder denervation procedures?

Bladder denervation procedures are designed to interrupt the nerve supply to the bladder. By interrupting the nerves that stimulate the bladder muscle to contract, the procedure can prevent bladder contractions. If the sensory fibers in the bladder are interrupted, this may also prevent bladder contractions because it prevents the bladder from sending messages to the central nervous system. These procedures may be reversible or permanent.

Reversible procedures

The simplest form of bladder denervation is **mucosal anesthesia**. An anesthetic is placed into the bladder that only affects the sensory fibers through the cysto-

Mucosal anesthesia

a type of procedure still being studied where an anesthetic agent is placed into the urethra, bladder, or rectum, to affect the sensory fibers in the bladder.

scope. If the patient responds to this procedure, it confirms that the problem is one of bladder sensation stimulating the overactivity. Local anesthesia can then be injected into the sacrum to block the sacral nerves supplying the bladder. Alternatively, a spinal anesthetic can be administered. How long the effects will last depends on the type of anesthestic used.

Permanent procedures

In individuals with an overactive bladder as a result of spinal cord injury, specialized spinal surgery to interrupt the nerves stimulating the bladder can be effective. However, if after this procedure the bladder fails to contract, the patient must empty his or her bladder by clean intermittent catheterization (CIC) (see Question 41).

Ingelman-Sundberg procedure

a transvaginal surgical technique that denerves the bladder to achieve control over uninhibited bladder contractions.

In females with refractory overactive bladder, a transvaginal procedure called the **Ingelman-Sundberg procedure** can be used. Prior to surgery the nerves that would be denervated by the procedure are injected with a local anesthetic. If the woman notes an improvement in her symptoms, the procedure is carried out. This procedure is done through the vagina.

PART FOUR

What Is Stress Urinary Incontinence?

What are the options for treatment for stress urinary incontinence?

How is someone with both stress and urge incontinence treated?

More ...

44. What is stress urinary incontinence?

As mentioned in Question 5, stress urinary incontinence is the involuntary loss of urine you experience when you exert yourself doing anything from sneezing or coughing to heavy lifting.

It occurs when the muscles in the pelvis that support the bladder and a part of the urethra (the proximal urethra) weaken. When you cough, laugh, or sneeze, the pressure in your abdomen increases. If the pelvic muscles supporting the bladder are weak, an increase in pressure in the abdomen pushes the bladder and proximal urethra out of the pelvis. As the bladder and proximal urethra are pushed out of their normal area increases in abdominal pressure are no longer transmitted equally to the bladder and urethra, and leakage may occur.

Stress urinary incontinence can affect women of all ages. Rarely, men can be affected with stress incontinence after procedures to treat both benign and cancerous enlargements of the prostate. About 20% of women between the ages of 20 to 65 years have stress urinary incontinence, and it is more common in women that have had children. Women with chronic obstructive pulmonary disease (COPD), women who have had prior pelvic surgery, and women with certain nerve-related problems are at increased risk of developing stress urinary incontinence.

45. Can someone have both stress and urge incontinence?

Yes. With both stress and urge incontinence, you would notice leakage associated with exertion (such as when coughing, laughing, or sneezing) as well as leakage associated with urgency. Typically, individuals who have both stress and urge incontinence are more bothered by the urge incontinence than the stress incontinence.

46. How is someone with both stress and urge incontinence treated?

As mentioned in the previous question, people with both stress and urge incontinence are often bothered more by the urge incontinence than the stress incontinence. Thus, most doctors will first treat the urge incontinence and associated urinary frequency. If the stress incontinence is still bothersome after treatment of the urge incontinence and urinary frequency, the stress incontinence will be treated as well. Options for treating stress urinary incontinence are discussed in Question 47.

47. What are the options for treatment for stress urinary incontinence?

The treatment options are surgery, behavioral therapy, and medication. Surgery is the main treatment for stress urinary incontinence. Behavioral therapy such as Kegel exercises (see Question 27) and/or medication may be helpful. Pessaries, a device placed into the vagina, and adhesive devices placed over the urethra, are also helpful in the management of stress incontinence.

There are a variety of surgical procedures for treating stress urinary incontinence. They vary from laparoscopic to minimally invasive to major abdominal surgery. The most common abdominal procedures are **"sling" procedures, tension-free vaginal tape (TVT) procedures**, and **transobturator tape (TOT) procedures**. All of these are designed to help support the urethra in order to prevent leakage. Cure rates are up to 90%, and at least 95% of patients note improvement. With sling, TVT, and TOT procedures there is a chance that you will have urinary retention (the

What Is Stress Urinary Incontinence?

Sling procedure
a surgical procedure used to treat stress incontinence which involves the use of a strip of natural or synthetic material placed under the urethra to act as a hammock.

Tension-free vaginal tape (TVT) procedure
a surgical procedure for treating stress urinary incontinence. In this procedure, a specialized tape is placed under the mid-urethra to support the bladder and urethra. (In a sling procedure, the tape is placed at a different location in the urethra.) An advantage of the TVT is that it may be performed under local anesthesia through a very small vaginal incision made right in the area of the mid-urethra.

Transobturator tape (TOT) procedure
a minimally invasive procedure for the treatment of stress urinary incontinence that works in the same way as the TVT but is placed differently.

inability to urinate). This requires that you use a catheter and possibly use clean intermittent catheterization (CIC) for a short time. (See Question 41 for a description of CIC.) Occasionally, correction of the urinary retention requires additional surgery.

There is no medication approved by the U.S. Food and Drug Administration (FDA) for treatment of stress urinary incontinence. However, there are medications that the FDA has approved for other uses that may improve symptoms of stress urinary incontinence. These medications include: topical estrogen cream, alpha-agonists, and tricyclic antidepressants.

Estrogen cream

Estrogen cream improves the health of the urethra and may help with urine leakage. To use it, you apply a dab of cream to the outside skin of the vagina, near the opening of the urethra. Your doctor will tell you how often you should apply it.

Alpha-agonists

Alpha-agonists are medications that cause muscles to tighten. They are often used when you have a cold with a runny nose. One commonly used alpha-agonist is pseudoephedrine (Sudafed). When used for stress urinary incontinence, alpha-agonists cause the muscle around the urethra to tighten, which in turn increases the pressure within the urethra. These medications can also cause tightening of the muscles around your arteries, which can cause your blood pressure to increase. It is best to check with your doctor before trying pseudoephedrine for stress incontinence.

Tricyclic antidepressants

Tricyclic antidepressants, such as amitriptyline (Elavil) and imipramine (Tofranil), are a special group of anti-depressants which have been found to work on the bladder and urethra. They relax the bladder muscle and thus lower the pressure in the bladder, and also tighten the muscle around the urethra, thereby increasing the urethral pressure. These medications may have side effects that affect the heart.

Several devices have been developed that "plug" the urethra in order to prevent leakage. All of the devices have to be applied directly onto or into the urethral opening. Some people find these devices helpful to use in particular situations, such as during a tennis game or when dancing, but often will not use the device on a daily basis because it requires removal and reapplica-tion/reinsertion every time you urinate.

Attempts have been made to provide more pressure in the urethra by injecting chemicals into the urethra (**intraurethral**) or around the urethra (**periurethral**). This type of therapy can only be used for a particular type of stress urinary incontinence. The procedure often can be performed in the doctor's office. It involves a **cystoscopy** (a procedure in which the blad-der and urethra are examined through a long, narrow, telescope-like device that is passed through the urethra into the bladder) and the injection of the material (called a bulking agent) through a long, slender needle into the urethra or around the urethra. There are cur-rently two chemicals that are approved for this use by the FDA: collagen (Contigen, Bard) and Duraspheres (Boston Scientific). The Zuidex system is composed of

Intraurethral
inside of the urethra.

Periurethral
around the urethra, outside of it.

Cytoscopy
a procedure in which the bladder and ure-thra are examined through a narrow, telescope-like device that is passed through the urethra into the bladder.

hyaluronic acid and a dextranomer copolymer gel is approved for use in stress urinary incontinence in Europe, but not currently available in the United States.

48. Does the same type of doctor treat OAB, urge incontinence, and stress urinary incontinence?

A urologist or urogynecologist can treat OAB, urge incontinence, and stress urinary incontinence. However, the first approach to treating OAB and urge incontinence is medication combined with behavioral therapy, so treatment often starts with the primary care provider. If medication and behavioral therapy do not work for you, then it is best to see a urologist or urogynecologist.

Surgery is the primary treatment for stress urinary incontinence, so it is often easiest to see a urologist or urogynecologist for treatment.

If you feel that you have both stress and urge incontinence, your primary care provider can start you on treatment for the urge incontinence and then refer you to a urologist or urogynecologist to treat the stress incontinence. Or, your doctor may refer you to a urologist or urogynecologist for treatment of both forms of incontinence.

PART FIVE

How Do I Select My Urologist or Urogynecologist?

Where can I find additional information about overactive bladder and urinary incontinence?

More ...

49. How do I select my urologist or urogynecologist?

Kathy's comment:

I was lucky to be working in urology. I knew many doctors in the field and it was fairly easy for me to make my decision. However, I think that you should get references from family and friends. It is also a great idea to ask nurses (if you know any) who work in the operating room (OR) with urologists. I think that a nurse can be your best identifier because she/he can evaluate skill level, etc.

Finding a **urologist** or **urogynecologist** to help you with your problem can be a challenge. Your primary care doctor, friends, and family may be able to help you to identify potential doctors. There are several things that you should consider when choosing your urologist or urogynecologist:.

1. Does this doctor perform the procedure regularly so that he/she maintains his/her surgical skills?

2. How many times has this doctor performed this procedure? What are his/her success and complication rates? It is perfectly okay to ask these questions and the urologist/urogynecologist should be comfortable answering them. Make sure that you ask the doctor for his/her specific success and complication rates. He/she may quote the results of large studies, but the doctors in the studies aren't the ones operating on you—it is the doctor that you are talking to who might perform the procedure.

3. Do you feel comfortable with the doctor?

4. Does your insurance company cover the procedure and the physician's costs?

Urologist

a physician who has completed a medical degree at a medical school as well as advanced training and practice in the field of urology, who is concerned with the study, diagnosis, and treatment of the genitourinary tract.

Urogynecologist

A specialty trained physician who has completed a medical degree at a medical school as well as advanced training and practice in the fields of urology, who is concerned with the study, diagnosis, and treatment of the genitourinary tract, and gynecology, the study, diagnosis, and treatment of the female genital tract, as well as endocrinology and the reproductive physiology of the female.

It is helpful to have a written list of questions ready before you meet with potential doctor(s). In addition to the questions listed here, you may want to keep a list of additional questions you would like to ask.

50. Where can I find additional information about overactive bladder and urinary incontinence?

Your local hospital may be able to provide you with information regarding nearby women's health centers, which will often have available information on overactive bladder and urinary incontinence. Other resources can be found in the Appendix that follows.

Laparoscopy

WHERE DOES THIS GO? A minimally invasive surgical procedure that allows a doctor to see the contents of the abdomen through the use of a specialized instrument. This instrument is attached to a light source, a fiberoptic camera, and surgical tools that are passed through small incisions under the umbilicus (belly button) and in other parts the abdomen.

Appendix

Several Web sites can be valuable resources for additional information regarding overactive bladder and urinary incontinence. They include:

www.overactivebladder.com

www.apta.org

www.medicalconsumerguide.com

www.niddk.nih.gov/health/urology/uibcw/index.htm

www.urologychannel.com/incontinence

www.mdlinx.com/patientlinx/index.cfm

www.bladdercontrol.com

www.drugs.com

www.kegel-exercises.com

www.nlm.nih.gov/medlineplus/urinaryincontinence.htm

www.medicinenet.com/urinaryincontinenceartivle.htm

www.lifebeyondthebathroom.com

The following book may be helpful:

The Urinary Incontinence Sourcebook, by Diane K. Newman and Mary K. Dzurinko. New York, NY: McGraw-Hill Co.; 1999.

Glossary

The following is a list of terms that appear in this book, or that may come up when you discuss your symptoms with your doctor.

Abscess: Collection of pus under the skin.

Acetylcholine: The neurotransmitter which when released from efferent parasympathetice nerves stimulates the bladder muscle to contract.

Acontractile bladder: A bladder that does not contract.

Afferent pathway: Messages (nerve impulse signals) inflowing to the central nervous system (brain and spinal cord) from the bladder.

Alpha-agonists: Type of medication that causes the muscles around the urethra (the sphincter muscles) to tighten or contract; may also cause tightening of the muscles that surround arteries and thus result in high blood pressure.

Angiocatheter: A small tube that is inserted into a blood vessel for injection of fluid. Dye is injected into it so that the surrounding blood vessels and cap-

illaries can be visualized to determine if there is a leak.

Antimuscarinic agent: A medication that blocks the effects of the neurotransmitter acetylcholine's action on muscarinic receptors. Muscarinic receptors in the bladder are involved in the control of bladder muscle contraction.

Atrophic vaginitis: A condition when a woman has thin, dry vaginal tissues do to little or no estrogen before or after menopause, or after hysterectomy and oophorectomy.

Autoaugmentation: A surgical procedure in which a part of the bladder muscle (the detrusor) is removed from the bladder leaving bladder lining (mucosa) behind to hold the urine.

Behaviorial therapy: A group of treatments designed for educating an individual about his/her medical condition so strategies can be developed to minimize or eliminate the symptoms.

Biofeedback: Information about one or more of an individual's normally unconscious body processes is made available to the individual through a visual (see), auditory (hear), or tactile (touch) signal.

Bladder augmentation: A surgical procedure whereby the bladder is enlarged with patches of organ tissue from the intestine (small or large), stomach, or ureter.

Bladder compliance: Describes the relationship between the change in bladder volume and change in bladder pressure.

Bladder denervation: Techniques to deaden or eliminate the nerves to the bladder in an effort to interrupt the nerve supply to the bladder and stop bladder contractions.

Bladder diary: Provides information on time of voiding and amount voided as well as incontinence episodes, pad usage/change in clothing, degree of leakage, and degree of urgency.

Bladder outlet: Area where the bladder joins the urethra.

Bladder sensation: During filling cystometry assessed as (1) first sensation of bladder filling, (2) first desire to void, and (3) strong desire to void.

Blood brain barrier (BBB): Semipermeable network of the tiniest blood vessels called capillaries with special endothelial cells surrounding the brain; the barrier prevents a variety of agents such as medications from passing through and entering the brain. Its function is to protect the brain from potentially harmful substances (like certain medications), other neurotransmitters, and hormones in the body, and to maintain the brain in a constant environment.

Botulinum neurotoxin: One of the most poisonous biologic chemicals known; produced by the bacterium *Clostridium botulinum;* very small amounts can lead to paralysis.

Capsaicin: The active ingredient found in chili peppers; inserted directly into the bladder to overstimulate the afferent nerves, and thus decrease bladder activity until the nerves regenerate neurotransmitters.

Catheter (Foley): A tubular instrument especially designed to be passed through the urethra into the bladder to drain the bladder.

Central nervous system: The brain and spinal cord; responsible for starting or preventing urination.

Chronic obstructive pulmonary disease (COPD): General term used for diseases with permanent or temporary narrowing of small bronchi in the lungs.

Chronic retention: Longstanding increased amount of urine in the bladder (postvoid residual). May be associated with urinary incontinence (overflow incontinence).

Clean intermittent catheterization (CIC): A type of temporary catheter to drain urine from the bladder on a regular basis throughout the day; usually self-accomplished by inserting the tube through the urethra into the bladder to empty the bladder. Most people are able to learn the procedure; it involves locating the urethral opening and being able to reach it to insert the catheter.

Cognition: General term encompassing thinking, learning, and memory.

Compliance: The consistency and accuracy with which a patient follows the treatment plan recommended by a physician or other healthcare professional.

Congenital: Existing at birth; refers to physical traits, conditions, diseases, anomalies, or malformations, etc., which may be either hereditary or because of an influence occurring during gestation up to the moment of birth.

Continence: Ability to hold urine and/or feces until a proper time for their discharge.

Cystocele: Hernia-like defect in women that occurs when the wall between the bladder and the vagina weakens, causing the bladder to drop or sag into the vagina.

Cystogram: X-ray test where radiographic fluid is inserted through a catheter placed into the bladder and x-rays are obtained. The contrast material causes the bladder to be "lit up" by the x-rays, so that the radiologist can see the area.

Cystoscope: A long telescope-like instrument that is passed through the urethra into the bladder for diagnostic and therapeutic purposes. It allows one to visualize inside the bladder and urethra.

Cystoscopy: A procedure in which the bladder and urethra are examined through a narrow telescope-like device that is passed through the urethra into the bladder for direct visualization of the bladder and urethral lining.

Darifenacin (Enablex, Novartis): An antimuscarinic agent recently approved for use in treatment of overactive bladder.

Deep vein thrombosis (DVT): A blood clot in the veins, usually in the legs, which can break off and go to the lungs/pulmonary embules.

Detrusor: The bladder muscle. Coordinated contraction of the detrusor and opening of the bladder outlet allows for normal urination.

Diverticula: Pouch or sac outpouching from a tubular or saccular organ such as the gut or bladder.

Duloxetine: A type of medication for stress urinary incontinence that is not yet approved by the FDA. Side effect: nausea.

Efferent pathway: Messages (nerve impulse signals) outflowing from the central nervous system to the peripheral nervous system.

Efficacy: Capacity or power to produce a desired effect.

Electromyography: Type of noninvasive test using skin patches to measure the activity in muscles.

Embolism: Obstruction or occlusion of a vessel by some tissue (blood clot) or air.

Enterocystoplasty: A surgical procedure to enlarge the bladder by the addition of a segment of small or large intestine.

Erosion: When the pubovaginal sling migrates from its position between the urethra and the vagina and relocates in one of the two organs.

Estrogens: A class of drugs, orally or topically applied, often used by primary care doctor and obstetrician/gynecologist.

Fascia: A sheet of connective tissue covering or binding together body structures.

Filling cystometrics (CMG): A component of the urodynamic study when the bladder is being filled and the pressures within the bladder are being measured along with an assessment of bladder sensation and bladder compliance.

Fistula: A communication between two organs; for example, a vesicovaginal fistula, whereby the bladder and vagina are connected by a small, open tract that allows urine to pass from the bladder into the vagina.

Fluoroscopy: Visualization of tissues and deep structures of the body by x-ray.

Frequency volume chart: A document plotting the amount of urine and number of times an individual urinates over a period of time.

Functional incontinence: A situation in which the bladder, urethra, and pelvic floor muscles are functioning properly, but physical or mental problems interferes with one's ability to independently get to the bathroom on time.

Gastrocystoplasty: Similar to enterocystoplasty, except that instead of using a piece of intestine, a segment of the stomach is used to patch the bladder.

Hematoma: A collection of blood that forms in a tissue, organ, or body space as a result of a broken blood vessel.

Hypertension: Transitory or sustained elevated arterial blood pressure. Untreated, it can cause cardiovascular damage.

Imipramine: An antidepressant medication used for overactive bladder; it has antimuscarinic properties and acts on two neurotransmitters in the brain (serotonin and noradrenaline) involved in the complex interactions related to normal bladder filling and emptying.

Incision: A cut; a surgical wound.

Ingelman-Sundberg procedure: A transvaginal surgical technique to deaden the nerves to the bladder to achieve control over involuntary bladder contractions.

Intraurethral: Inside of the urethra.

Intravesical: Inside the bladder.

Kegel exercises: Exercises designed to strengthen weak pelvic floor muscles.

Laparoscopy: A minimally invasive surgical procedure that allows a doctor to see the contents of the abdomen through the use of a specialized instrument. This instrument is attached to a light source, a fiberoptic camera, and surgical tools that are passed through small incisions under the umbilicus (belly button) and in other parts of the abdomen.

Local anesthesia: A short-acting spinal anesthetic or anesthesia applied locally.

Lower urinary tract symptoms (LUTS): Term used to describe symptoms associated with storage and emptying of the bladder.

Micturition: The action of voiding urine.

Mixed urinary incontinence: Involuntary leakage of urine associated with urgency as well as with exertion, effort, sneezing, or coughing. The combination of urgency incontinence and stress urinary incontinence.

Mucosa: A mucous tissue lining various tubular structures, including the bladder and urethra.

Mucosal anesthesia: A type of procedure still being studied where an anesthetic agent is placed into the urethra, bladder, or rectum, to affect the sensory fibers in the bladder. In theory, if the patient responds to this procedure, it would confirm that the problem is one of bladder sensation stimulating the overactivity.

Muscarinic receptor: A membrane-bound protein that contains a recognition site for acetylcholine; a combination of acetylcholine with the receptor initiates a physiologic change (i.e., slowing of the heart rate, increased glandular activity, and stimulation of smooth muscle contractions).

Neuromodulation: Surgical placement of a permanent continuous nerve stimulator and its electrode wires.

Nocturia: The complaint that the individual has to wake at night one or more times to void.

Obstruction: Outflow of urine from the bladder is blocked; may be caused by prostate enlargement or urethral strictures, narrowed areas in the urethra, or medications that affect the function of the urethra, among others.

Orthostatic hypotension: Lowering of blood pressure while moving from a sitting to a standing position.

Overactive bladder: Urgency, with or without urgency incontinence, usually with frequency and nocturia.

Oxybutynin: One of the oldest pharmaceutical therapies for overactive bladder. It is effective, but its use is limited by a high incidence of side effects, including dry mouth and constipation.

Oxybutynin extended release (Ditropan XL, J&J): A type of pharmaceutical therapy for overactive bladder. It is similar to oxybutynin, but is a sustained release formulation with less dry mouth and constipation than oxybutynin.

Pelvic floor muscles: A group of muscles that form a sling or hammock across the outlet of the pelvis; these muscles, together with their surrounding tissue, are responsible for keeping all of the pelvic organs (bladder, uterus, and rectum) in place and functioning correctly.

Pelvic organ prolapse: A weakening in the pelvic floor support structures (muscles and fascia) that allows pelvic organs to drop into the vaginal space. May cause visible or palpable bulge at vaginal opening. Can involve bladder, uterus, small bowel or rectum.

Perineum: Area between the thighs extending from the tail bone (coccyx) to the pubis (between the vulva and anus in the female and scrotum and anus in the male) and lying below the pelvic diaphragm.

Peripheral nervous system: Nerves connecting in the body other than the brain and spinal cord; responsible for the coordination of bladder contraction and urethral relaxation during normal voiding.

Periurethral: Around the urethra, outside of it.

Periurethral injection: A type of shot where a needle filled with the agent to be injected is inserted alongside the urethra and the material injected. May be used in the treatment of Type III SUI.

Poor contractility: Where the bladder muscle cannot generate and/or sustain a contraction that completely empties it of urine; may result from damage to the nerves supplying the bladder (spinal cord injury or conditions like spina bifida), chronic overdistention of the bladder, severe long-term blockages of the outlet, or medications.

Poorly compliant bladder: Holds urine at higher than normal bladder pressures, causing poor emptying of the kidneys, a backup of urine in the kidneys, and eventually kidney damage.

Postprostatectomy urinary incontinence: Leakage of urine in men who have had a radical prostatectomy; in most cases, this resolves after the pelvic muscles heal.

Postvoid residual urine: The amount of urine left in the bladder after urinating; if elevated may lead to urinary tract infections, bladder stones, and further distention of the bladder, leading to poor bladder contractility.

Potty training: Ability of toddlers to learn how to hold their urine and then voluntarily empty the bladder at a socially acceptable time. The process involves maturity as the brain develops a communication network with the bladder.

Pressure flow study: A specialized study used to assess whether there is any obstruction to the outflow of urine.

Probanthine bromide: A nonselective antimuscarinic medication for overactive bladder; individual doses will vary.

Prolapse: The lack of support with respect to the floor and the ceiling of the vagina; this scaffolding that supports the vagina also supports other structures such as the bladder, the uterus, and the rectum. If these organs are not well supported, they may descend/herniate into the vagina.

Pubovaginal sling: Type of surgical procedure that uses a synthetic or fascial sling that is placed under the proximal urethra to support the bladder neck and proximal urethra.

Radical prostatectomy: A procedure performed for prostate cancer. Includes removal of the prostate, seminal vesicles, and part of the vas deferens.

Resiniferatoxin: A chemical derived from a cactus-like plant, *Euphorbia resinifera*; inserted directly into the bladder to overstimulate the afferent nerves, and thereby decrease bladder activity until the nerves regenerate neurotransmitters.

Sacrum: Refers to the large, irregular, triangular-shaped bone made up of the five fused vertebrae below the lumbar region; comprises part of the pelvis.

Skin patch electrodes: A noninvasive, no-pain method used in testing muscle activity or pressures involving a flat adhesive patch with embedded wires.

Sling procedure: A surgical procedure used to treat stress incontinence which involves the use of a strip of natural or synthetic material placed under the urethra to act as a hammock.

Small capacity bladder: Organ cannot hold much urine because of fibrosis or scarring or neurologic causes; the bladder loses its elasticity so the individual must urinate more frequently.

Solifenacin: (Vesicare, Yamanouchi) An antimuscarinic medication recently approved by the FDA for use in overactive bladder.

Sphincter mechanism: The muscular mechanism that helps maintain continence of urine and stool.

Stasis: When there is high pressure in the bladder, the ureter is unable to push the urine into the bladder, causing a backup of urine within the ureter and eventually the kidneys.

Stress urinary incontinence: (also known as genuine stress urinary incontinence, GSUI) Involuntary loss of bladder control during periods of increased abdominal pressure such as coughing, laughing, heavy lifting, or straining.

Suprapubic tube: A type of tube placed directly into the bladder at the time of surgery that exits through the skin on your lower abdomen to drain the bladder; less irritating than a Foley catheter.

Tension-free vaginal tape (TVT) procedure: A surgical procedure for treating stress urinary incontinence. In this procedure, a specialized tape is placed under the mid-urethra to support the bladder and urethra. (In a sling procedure, the tape is placed at a different location in the urethra.)

An advantage of the TVT is that it may be performed under local anesthesia through a very small vaginal incision made right in the area of the mid-urethra.

Timed voiding: A type of behavioral therapy that involves urinating at two- to three-hour intervals, no matter if there is a desire to urinate or not.

Tissue engineering: A pioneering technique of growing cells designed to mimic the behavior and reproducibility of normal cells.

Tolterodine: First antimuscarinic drug that was developed solely for use in overactive bladder.

Tolterodine, Pfizer (Detrol LA): Type of antimuscarinic drug developed in a capsule containing small microspheres that are released slowly into the body, allowing for a sustained release of medication; used for overactive bladder and has a lower incidence of side effects.

Transcutaneous: Denotes the passage of substances through the unbroken skin.

Transdermal: Medication is delivered to the body by a skin patch.

Transdermal oxybutynin (Oxytrol, Watson): A patch formulation of oxybutynin that is changed twice a week. The patch delivers 3.9 mg of oxybutynin per day.

Transient (temporary) incontinence: Leakage of urine caused by illness or medications that interferes with normal bladder function. Treatment of underlying cause should resolve incontinence.

Transobturator tape (TOT) procedure: A minimally invasive procedure for the treatment of stress urinary incontinence.

Transurethral injection: A type of shot where a cystoscope is inserted into the urethra and a thin, long needle is advanced through the cystoscope, into the urethra; the chemical is then injected into the urethra to treat Type III SUI.

Transurethral prostatectomy (TURP): Removal of the prostate through the urethra.

Tricyclic antidepressants: A class of medications which may be used to treat incontinence. They lower the bladder pressure by relaxing the bladder muscle and also help further by tightening the sphincter muscle.

Trospium chloride (Sanctura, Inderus): An antimuscarinic medication for overactive bladder that has been recently approved for use in the United States by the FDA.

Ultrasound: A noninvasive test using radiowaves (frequency greater than 30,000 MHz); used to evaluate the kidneys and bladder to assess bladder emptying capacity.

Ureter: A long, thin, hollow tube that connects the kidneys to the bladder so that urine can pass out of the kidney and into the bladder.

Ureterocystoplasty: Technique that is used in patients who have a dilated distal ureter, which can be isolated, opened, and used as a bladder patch.

Urethra: Canal leading from the bladder to outside of the body to allow for passage of urine. In the female, it is ~4 cm long and opens in the perineum between the clitoris and vaginal opening; in the male it is ~20 cm long and opens in the glans penis.

Urethral sphincter: A muscle that when contracted closes the urethra.

Urgency incontinence: Unintended leakage or loss of urine into clothing or bedclothes as a result of an involuntary detrusor contraction.

Urinalysis: A type of test of the urine to determine normalcy or abnormality.

Urinary frequency: Having to void more than eight times per day with normal intake of fluids.

Urinary incontinence: Involuntary loss of urine. May be the result of an overactive bladder, stress incontinence, functional incontinence, or other causes.

Urinary retention: The inability to empty bladder completely. Acute urinary retention is the total inability to urinate.

Urinary urgency: Sudden compelling desire to urinate that often is difficult to defer.

Urine cytology: A small amount of urine is sent to the pathologist, who examines the urine sample to determine the presence or absence of any cancer cells.

Urodynamic study: A special test used to determine how the bladder and urethral muscles work; includes measuring storage and emptying of the bladder.

Uroflow: The rate of flow of the urine stream; often a component of a

urodynamic study, but may be performed in the office.

Urogynecologist: A specialty trained physician who has completed a medical degree at a medical school as well as advanced training in the field of obstetrics/gynecology and subsequent additional training in a pelvic-floor medicine.

Urologist: A physician who has completed a medical degree at a medical school as well as advanced training and practice in the field of urology, the study, diagnosis, and treatment of the genitourinary tract. Some urologists may pursue additional training in pelvic floor medicine.

Urothelium: The inner lining of the urinary tract (kidneys, ureter, bladder).

Uterine prolapse: When the uterus is not supported by the pelvic floor and sinks down into vaginal space.

Valsalva leak point pressure: The intra-abdominal pressure generated by a Valsalva maneuver that results in urinary leakage.

Valsalva maneuver: Any forced expiratory effort ("strain") against a closed airway; used to study cardiovascular effects as well as poststrain responses.

Vesicoureteral reflux: Urine passing backwards from the bladder into ureters and may go all the way to the kidneys.

Videourodynamics: Use of intermittent fluoroscopy (taking x-ray pictures) during the urodynamic study to visualize the bladder and urethra.

Void: To evacuate urine and/or feces.

Index

Index